Personal Care for People Who Care

10th Edition

Your Guide to Choosing Cruelty-Free
Cosmetics, Household, Personal Care
and Companion Animal Products.

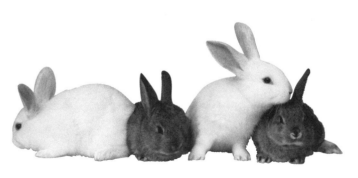

A Publication of The National Anti-Vivisection Society
Chicago, Illinois

Personal Care for People Who Care
10th Edition

Personal Care for People Who Care is a publication of The National Anti-Vivisection Society (NAVS), a national not-for-profit educational organization. NAVS promotes greater compassion, respect and justice for animals through educational programs based on respected ethical and scientific theory and supported by extensive documentation of the cruelty and waste of vivisection. NAVS' educational programs are directed at increasing public awareness about vivisection, identifying humane solutions to human problems, developing alternatives to the use of animals, and working with like-minded individuals and groups to effect changes which help to end the suffering of innocent animals.

The information provided in this book is based on the most current data available at the time of publication. For the most up-to-date information, contact the company directly.

Please recycle this book.

ISBN 1-888635-02-9   ✪ Printed on recycled paper.

TABLE OF CONTENTS

Cruelty-Free Shopping Made Easy

As a caring and compassionate individual, ensuring the safety and well-being of the animals with whom you share your life is no doubt very important to you. *Personal Care for People Who Care* is an opportunity to show your concern for the many animals whom you don't know, but who nonetheless need your help.

You may already know about the suffering of animals used to test products and ingredients in the name of human safety. Rabbits, mice, rats and guinea pigs suffer needlessly in laboratories and research facilities across the United States. Millions of animals have been the subjects of painful tests routinely performed as part of the complex development of most new and "improved" cosmetics, personal care items and household products on their way to store shelves.

This 10th edition of *Personal Care for People Who Care* is about progress and about hope. With encouragement from caring consumers, more and more *major* companies are pledging to end animal testing, putting their convictions into practice through incremental adoption of non-animal alternatives. Many of these companies are funding the research for development and validation of these alternatives (see page 15). Fewer companies than ever before now claim that they must test their products and ingredients on animals to ensure their safety. And many more companies are acknowledging that a vast majority of the animal tests they once conducted are not necessary to protect human health and safety.

> *Vivisection: the act of cutting into, dissecting or harming the body of an animal, especially for the purpose of product testing, dissection or scientific research.*

By adopting a cruelty-free lifestyle, one that chooses respect for animals in selecting personal care, cosmetic, household and companion animal products, you are making a positive statement to companies selling these products. For

> *Cruelty free: product testing policy of a company that prohibits the use of animals to test its ingredients and/or final products. This includes not purchasing animal-tested ingredients from outside suppliers.*

anyone concerned about respect, compassion and justice for animals, purchasing products that are not animal-tested is a simple and convenient way to match your money to your convictions, while sending a powerful message to companies that you won't support an industry that perpetuates animal suffering.

To help you choose cruelty-free products, the National Anti-Vivisection Society (NAVS) has prepared this comprehensive guide to companies that do and do not test their products and/or ingredients on animals. It also lists health-based charities that do and do not fund animal-based research—an important consideration as you decide which organizations to support in your everyday gift-giving as well as estate planning.

NAVS is a national, not-for-profit educational organization dedicated to ending animal suffering through positive and effective programs that help educate people about the cruelty and waste of animal experimentation. We also support passage of animal protection legislation and fund the development of alternatives to the use of animals in research.

Personal Care for People Who Care makes it simple and convenient for you to put compassion at the top of your shopping list...and make a real difference in the lives of animals.

How to Use This Book

Personal Care for People Who Care is the most comprehensive guide available to use when shopping for cruelty-free personal care, cosmetics, household and companion animal products. All of the information provided is supplied to us directly from each company.

The principal part of this book includes two main sections: those companies that <u>did</u> respond to our questionnaire and those that <u>did not</u>. For companies that did respond to our inquiries, each directory listing will contain one of these symbols before the name of the company:

♥ means that this company **DOES NOT** test *final products* or *ingredients* on animals, nor do any of its outside suppliers. Therefore, the company is cruelty free. (Suppliers are separate companies that manufacture or provide ingredients that are used to make the final products.)

🐾 means that while the parent company does test on animals, this individual subsidiary/division **does not** test *final products* or *ingredients* on animals.

◆ means that while the company **does not** test its *final products* or *ingredients* on animals, it has no agreement with its suppliers stating that they do not test their ingredients on animals.

▼ means that this company **DOES** test *final products* and/or *ingredients* on animals.

Use the inside back flap as a handy reference guide to the symbols utilized in this book. It's also a great way to hold your place while you're shopping!

You will also find one or more symbols after the name of the company:

※ means that the company does not use any animal-derived ingredients in its products.

■ means that the company is a *manufacturer*.

● means that the company is a *distributor*.

⊡ means that the company is a *mail-order company*.

Easy to Use Special Features

✔ New in this edition is a convenient mail-order section of cruelty-free companies for individuals who do not have easy access to cruelty-free products. See page 173 for a listing of companies that provide mail-order service.

✔ Also included is an expanded section on parent companies, their subsidiaries, and individual brand names. This information will help you untangle the corporate maze and identify who owns what! See page 139 for a listing of these companies.

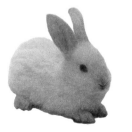

Have Decades of Advocacy Begun To Pay Off?

This edition of *Personal Care for People Who Care* is about **progress.** It's about major manufacturers of personal care and household products that have made giant strides in reducing and even eliminating animal testing. We applaud their efforts and we congratulate all who have worked hard to encourage companies to stop animal testing.

In the 9th edition, we were pleased to include Gillette as a cruelty-free company for the first time. In this 10th edition we considered including Colgate-Palmolive, Procter & Gamble and many other companies as non-testers, but they didn't yet qualify according to our strict criteria for cruelty-free companies. But the fact that we could even consider such an action is an indication of how far these large corporations have progressed, collectively decreasing their reliance on animal testing.

Procter & Gamble, Colgate-Palmolive and Bristol-Myers Squibb have all come forward with strong positive statements concerning their commitment to end animal testing when viable non-animal alternatives can be used.

A sample of these major companies and their stated policies regarding animal testing are listed below:

Alberto-Culver: Does not conduct animal testing on any products whose ingredients or formulas have already met their safety criteria. This includes more than 96% of personal care products and 100% of grocery products. They do conduct limited animal tests on new formulations or technologies that come in contact with the skin or eyes or could be accidently ingested.

Bristol-Myers Squibb: For over ten years has had a program to reduce their reliance on animal testing methods. They do not test their finished products, including cosmetics, on animals. Nor do they contract out such testing. This is also true for nearly all of their consumer product ingredients. As a matter of policy, their scientists must consider the use of *in vitro* methods wherever feasible.

Church & Dwight: Avoids animal testing whenever complete and satisfactory information exists to show that products are safe. They have experienced considerable success in avoiding animal testing through this practice, especially on their consumer products.

Even a Little Is Too Much

Companies that test some of their products or ingredients on animals are designated as "testers," even if only a small portion of their products are still tested. However, subsidiaries or divisions of a testing company may receive a separate designation (❦) if we receive independent confirmation that the subsidiary or division does not conduct any animal testing on their own products. Those products would also receive the ❦ designation. For more information on parent companies and subsidiaries and brand names, see page 139.

Colgate-Palmolive: Declared a voluntary moratorium on animal testing of their personal care products designed for adults and the ingredients used in those products. [**NAVS Note:** This moratorium, however, applies to only 98% of their personal care products. The company has failed to specify which products are still tested and which are not, therefore all of their products are designated as "tested."] The company's worldwide policy is that they are committed to the objectives of further reducing and indeed ultimately eliminating the need for animal testing.

Gillette: Since 1996, no laboratory animals were used to test Gillette personal care or other consumer products or ingredients.

Johnson & Johnson: New compounds receive full safety testing, including the use of lab animals. The company does not, however, conduct the LD-50 test and uses as few animals as possible for tests they do perform. For instance, ingredients in Neutrogena products have been proven safe historically, so instead of using laboratory animals to assess the safety of its formulations, the company performs a number of predictive tests on humans volunteers.

Procter & Gamble: Committed to the ultimate elimination of animal testing. They no longer use animals in evaluating the safety of non-food, non-drug consumer product formulations. They will adopt new alternative methods as soon as they are scientifically and, when necessary, legally accepted.

SmithKline Beecham: Conducts animal tests only when they are developing new products using new ingredients whose safety has not been established. Then, animal tests would only be undertaken after a comprehensive internal review is conducted on the benefits of conducting such tests. They have discontinued use of the LD-50 test.

In addition, each of these companies has funded significant research into alternatives to animal testing, either in-house or through such groups as the Johns Hopkins Center for Alternatives to Animal Testing (CAAT).

Even with these significant advances, the National Anti-Vivisection Society, in rating whether companies are cruelty free, determined that when any animal testing continues companies cannot be considered "cruelty free." Some companies have dramatically reduced their reliance on animal testing, which is a positive change in policy. However, as long as any animal testing continues, these companies have not yet earned the cruelty-free designation.

We applaud the commitment on the part of large corporations to ultimately end the use of any animal testing and strongly encourage the further development of viable non-animal alternatives.

The European Union passed a resolution several years ago to ban testing on cosmetics within Europe. This was to first take effect in 1998, then in 1999, but it has again been postponed. Hopefully this policy will take effect in the year 2000. The reason given for the delay is that sufficient validated alternatives are not yet available to abandon animal testing altogether. Great Britain, however, has already banned animal testing on cosmetics and its parliament deserves kudos for its progressive leadership on this issue.

Although much progress has been made, there is still much to accomplish in the development—and just as importantly, the validation and implementation—of non-animal alternative tests by both industry and by government regulatory agencies. With ongoing cooperation and commitment among animal advocates, industry and the government, progress will continue to be made on behalf of the animals.

What Is Animal Testing?

Annually, millions of animals have been exposed to tests on personal care, cosmetics and household products. Rabbits, guinea pigs, rats and mice have been forced to ingest harmful substances, or have caustic ingredients rubbed on their exposed skin or in their eyes. Then these animals are killed.

While fewer animals are used in the development of products than five years ago, there are two tests that continue to be utilized by companies that still test on animals. These outmoded tests have been used for decades, testing the same chemicals on the same types of animals year after year, despite the fact that the information resulting from these tests is not being used to protect human safety but only to determine levels of toxicity. Furthermore, there are more reliable and less expensive non-animal alternatives available. Following is a description of the two most common tests, the Draize and the LD-50.

The Draize Test

The Draize test attempts to measure the harmfulness of chemicals by observing the damage they cause to the eyes and skin of animals. In the Draize test for *eye irritancy,* solutions of products are applied directly into the eyes of groups of conscious animals.

In the Draize test for *skin irritancy,* the test substances are applied to shaved and abraded skin. (Skin is abraded by firmly pressing adhesive tape onto the animal's body and quickly stripping it off. The process is repeated until several layers of skin have been exposed.)

During the test period, which usually lasts at least several days, the animals can suffer extreme pain. The eye irritancy test compounds often cause irreparable damage to the animals' eyes, leaving them ulcerated and bleeding. At the end of the test period, all of the animals are killed in order to determine the effects of the tested substances on internal organs.

The LD-50 Test

The LD-50 test is used to measure the acute toxicity levels of certain ingredients on live animals. LD-50 stands for Lethal Dose 50 Percent—the amount or concentration of a substance that will kill half of a test group of animals within a specified time period when that substance is forcibly ingested, inhaled or otherwise exposed to an animal. During the test period, the animals typically suffer acute distress—pain, convulsions, discharge, diarrhea and bleeding from the eyes and mouth. At the end of the test period, those animals who have not already died are killed.

Long known to be poor predictors of human health, the LD-50 and Draize tests have been shown to be less reliable and more expensive than existing non-animal alternatives. There are many variables among species of animals and even among individual animals. The results of non-animal tests tend to be more consistent and better predictors for human reactions. In addition, companies are spared the expense of breeding, caging, feeding and disposing of animals that are used in testing laboratories. Companies are taking a closer look at animal tests and the results. Many major companies are discontinuing the use of these tests on products and ingredients that have already been tested or for which the information is otherwise available.

Databases of information on chemical interactions and toxicity levels also contribute greatly to a reduction in animal testing. With the continued development of alternatives, animal tests, like the slide rule, will someday be made obsolete by advancements in technology.

When Do Government Regulations Require Animal Tests?

The U.S. Food and Drug Administration (FDA) requires intensive testing of **pharmaceutical products (drugs)** and a number of chemical compounds that change the chemistry of the body when used. At this time, the FDA requires some of that testing to be carried out on animals. This requirement has been successfully challenged by personal care manufacturer Tom's of Maine, which received approval for its fluoride toothpaste (fluoride is a chemical required to be tested by the FDA), without the use of animals. It can be done.

Progress has been made in requiring government agencies, including the FDA and the Environmental Protection Agency (EPA), to consider non-animal alternatives to satisfy their health and safety requirements. Industry, animal advocates and members of the scientific community are working together to encourage the development and validation of more non-animal alternatives in the coming years.

What Are the Alternatives to Animal Testing?

Thanks to advancements in modern technology and a growing number of scientists seeking a better way, there are non-animal methods for testing products currently in use—and more are being developed every year. These safe, innovative and reliable alternatives are not only saving animals' lives, they often provide the necessary data in a shorter time and at less cost than the traditional animal tests.

After a new test is developed, it must go through a rigorous validation process before results from the test are regarded as reliable for general use. This process involves review and hearings by experts through the National Toxicology Program Interagency Center for the Evaluation of Alternative Toxicological Methods (NICEATM) and the Interagency Coordinating Committee on the Validation of Alternative Methods (ICCVAM).

What Are the 3 "Rs?"

Within the scientific community, the generally accepted definition of "alternatives" was established in 1959 by William M.S. Russell & R.L Burch in their publication, *The Principles of Humane Experimental Technique*. This philosophy is characterized by the three "Rs":

• Refinement—improvement that minimizes the pain, suffering and stress of animals used in research;

• Reduction—a decrease in the number of animals used while enhancing the quality and yield of information; and

• Replacement—scientifically valid substitutions for current live animal methodologies.

The validation and regulatory acceptance of alternative tests is critical to the adoption of more humane scientific methodologies.

Although scientists have concluded that no single non-animal alternative thus far developed can completely replace animal tests like the Draize test, companies are able to avoid animal testing by relying on a battery of non-animal alternatives, including in vitro (test tube) technology. They also refer to the U.S. GRAS (Generally Regarded As Safe), a list of thousands of ingredients already known to be safe, as well as information on historical use and chemical structure. Human clinical studies are also a valuable and accepted means of testing products, especially for biomedical and medical device testing.

Some of the most commonly used non-animal product safety tests include:

• Agarose Diffusion Method, which is used to determine the toxicity of plastics and other synthetic materials used in medical devices. In this test, human cells and a small amount of test material are placed in a container and separated by a thin layer of agarose, a derivative of the sea plant agar. If the test material is an irritant, a zone of killed cells appears around the substance.

• Computer and Mathematical Models, which predict the irritancy of test substances on the basis of physical and chemical structures and properties.

• EpiDerm, which uses neonatal foreskin-derived normal skin cells grown into 3-dimensional tissue for dermal irritancy testing, percutaneous absorption studies and basic skin research.

• EpiOcular, which uses an artificial tissue manufactured like EpiDerm, but which is more similar to the cornea, the outermost covering of the eye.

- Epipack Test, which uses sheets of cloned human skin cells to estimate a human's reaction to a skin irritant.

- Irritection Assay, which uses a protein alteration system to assess irritancy. Changes in the protein matrix caused by foreign materials are indicative of potential irritation of eye or skin tissue.

- Neutral Red Bioassay, in which neutral red, a water-soluble dye, is added to normal human skin cells in a 96-well tissue culture plate. A computer measurement of the level of uptake of the dye by the cells is used to indicate relative toxicity, eliminating observer bias.

- Transepithelial Passage Assay, which measures the chemical-induced changes in an artificial barrier layer constructed of human (in some cases animal) cells to estimate the eye irritation potential of chemicals.

The following non-animal based test has recently been declared valid by ICCVAM:

- Corrositex Assay, for use in evaluating the corrosivity or burn potential of certain classes of chemicals, uses a collagen matrix barrier as a kind of artificial skin and pH indicator dyes to detect how long it takes a chemical to penetrate this barrier.

The following alternatives, while they may use **animal parts** or **cells** as part of the test, **significantly reduce** the number of live animals currently used to test toxicity.

- 3T3 NRU PT is a cytotoxicity test in which mouse-derived cells are exposed both to test chemicals and to visible light to measure the phototoxic potential of chemicals.

• Bovine Corneal Opacity and Permeability Asssay (BCOP), which uses bovine corneas obtained as a by-product of normal slaughter-house procedures to measure direct opacity and permeability to fluorescein, reflecting damage to corneal epithelium.

• Chorioallantoic Membrane (CAM) Test, which uses fertilized chicken eggs to evaluate eye irritancy by observing the reaction of the chorioallantoic membrane to test substances.

The following alternatives may use **whole animals** as part of the test or to provide tissue each time the test is run. However they **reduce** the number of animals used or **lessen the amount of suffering** of the animals as opposed to the normal animal test that they replace. These alternatives are examples of "reduction" or "refinement" tests, not "replacements" for animals in testing altogether.

• Frog Embryo Teratogenesis Assay (FETAX), which uses frog embryos to evaluate the developmental toxicity potential of chemicals.

• Local Lymph Node Assay, which can be used for assessing the allergic contact dermatitis potential of chemicals. This replaces existing guinea pig tests with tests on mice and reduces the number of animals used and the time taken to perform the test. This has already been validated by ICCVAM.

• Rat Skin Transcutaneas Electrical Resistance (TER), which uses skin discs taken from the pelts of young rats to predict the corrosivity potential of chemicals.

Questions About Animal Testing

Q. Are companies required by the federal government to test their products on animals?

A. Many people believe that testing cosmetics on animals is required by law, but that's not the case. The Federal Food, Drug and Cosmetic Act does not require cosmetic manufacturers or marketers to test their products on animals for safety. In fact, the Food and Drug Administration (FDA) actually encourages the use of testing techniques that do not use whole living animals. At the same time, however, the FDA strongly urges cosmetic manufacturers to conduct whatever toxicological tests are appropriate to substantiate the safety of their cosmetics.

Cosmetics and personal care products which are also intended to treat or prevent disease, or which affect the structure or functions of the human body, are considered "drugs." These products must comply with the drug testing requirements of the FDA, and animals are always used as test models. Examples of these products include:

- Suntan preparations intended to protect against sunburn
- Deodorants that are also antiperspirants
- Anti-dandruff shampoos
- Topical acne medication

The government, through the FDA, mandates that all drugs be tested on animals. This is current law. That is why *Personal Care for People Who Care* focuses on those categories where manufacturers have an option when determining the toxicity levels and safety of a product.

Q. Is animal testing necessary to protect consumers?

A. No. An abundance of evidence proves that animal testing contributes little or nothing to consumer safety, nor does it provide information for the effective treatment of injuries that may result from the use or misuse of the product. In fact, testing on animals cannot accurately predict an allergic reaction in some humans. And some products that have been found to be safe in animals have caused serious side effects in people. Simply put, testing an ingredient or product on an animal does not make it safe. In fact, products that **have** been tested on animals and which can cause serious injury or death are side-by-side on shelves with other products that are safe for consumers and yet have not been tested on animals.

Q. If products are tested on animals for human safety, why are many household products still labelled as "hazardous?"

A. Animal testing does not assure that products are safe. Animal testing merely determines the level of toxicity. Although companies claim that they test products on animals to substantiate their safety, products which have been tested on animals, such as permanent wave solutions and oven cleaners, are regularly introduced into the marketplace even though they are toxic. That's because no amount of animal testing can change the fact that many of these products are harmful if ingested or used in a way not intended by the manufacturer. The manufacturer must still label the product as "hazardous" when it's sold.

Q. Do vitamins have to be tested on animals?

A. The FDA does not require companies to test vitamins on animals, nor does it require FDA registration of vitamins. The FDA's main concern is that the vitamins are correctly labeled for their contents, which can be confirmed using chemical rather than animal tests. The FDA would only animal-test a vitamin if the agency suspected that it contained a toxic agent.

Q. Why are so many contact lens products tested on animals?
A. Contact lenses and lens care products are considered medical devices, not pharmaceuticals. Although the FDA has not published any regulations requiring animal testing of contact lenses or lens care products, the agency has made testing guidance documents available to manufacturers. These documents do not carry the weight of regulations, but they do recommend preclinical testing on animals. Manufacturers choosing to use alternative procedures must provide documentation explaining why an alternate test procedure is an acceptable substitute. "Acceptable" means that it has been validated and accepted by the scientific community.

Q. If a company is not listed in the book, or is listed in the "did not respond" section, is it fair to assume that they test on animals?
A. No. Please do not make the assumption that those companies that did not respond to NAVS' inquiries use animals for testing. It simply means that these companies chose not to provide us with information regarding their testing policies.

Q. Why are some companies that claim not to test on animals listed in *Personal Care* as testing?
A. In the 10th edition of *Personal Care* we have added a new symbol, ❧, to indicate subsidiaries and their products that are cruelty free, even though their parent company tests.

There are some subsidiaries, such as Neutrogena (which is owned by Johnson & Johnson—a tester), which have traditionally not tested their products or ingredients on animals. However, when these subsidiaries are owned by a parent company that does conduct some animal testing, its status is in question. In the past, these subsidiaries would have received the same testing designation as their parent, even if they did not themselves test their products or ingredients. In order to provide consumers with more specific information, we apply the new designation (🐾) when we receive independent documentation of a subsidiary's cruelty-free policies. See page 139 for details of parent companies and their subsidiaries/divisions.

Q. Where can I find cruelty-free products?
A. Just about anywhere you normally shop! Look for cruelty-free products in your local supermarket and department stores, pharmacies and health food stores. If you don't see cruelty-free products at a particular store, encourage the store manager to carry these items. Many cruelty-free products are also available through the mail. A special section has been added to help you find mail-order items that are cruelty free (see page 173).

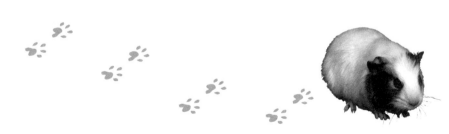

What Can You Do to Help?

One of the best ways to help end the practice of animal testing is to shop cruelty free, using *Personal Care for People Who Care* as a guide. Show your compassion by selecting only those products that have not been animal tested. When you buy cruelty free, you're making a powerful economic statement to those companies that still test their products or ingredients on animals.

But don't stop there! The animals need your help. Here are some other ways you can make a real difference for animals.

☑ **Take this book with you whenever you shop.** It will help you make the cruelty-free choice every time.

☑ **Give this book as a gift.** Your friends will appreciate your thoughtful gesture in helping them learn more about the issue of animal experimentation and how to become a more compassionate consumer.

☑ **Spread the word about cruelty-free living.** Encourage store owners to carry *Personal Care for People Who Care,* and order additional copies of this book to donate to your local library and school.

☑ **Write letters to companies that still test on animals.** Corporations are very concerned about their public image, and your polite but firm message, written from your heart, can have a powerful impact.

☑ **Contact your local newspapers and radio stations.** Tell them you're concerned about society's treatment of animals and request that they run more stories about this important issue. You may also want to have them call NAVS and request our radio public service announcements.

☑ **Become a more informed animal advocate and consumer.** Find out more about the cruelty and waste of product testing, and share that information with friends, family and co-workers. NAVS has a number of publications available. See page 195 for details.

☑ **Don't invest in the stock of companies that test their products on animals.** If you already hold securities in any of these companies, use your power as a shareholder to encourage a change in policy.

☑ **Appeal to legislators.** Inform your elected representatives about product testing on animals. Encourage them to support legislation to implement alternative methods of ensuring product safety.

☑ **Donate your charitable dollars to organizations that don't fund animal research.** See pages 25-31 for a listing of health-based charities that do and do not support animal research.

☑ **Visit the NAVS web site at www.navs.org.** Find out more about animal experimentation and how you can help end animal suffering.

☑ **Join the National Anti-Vivisection Society.** We'll keep you informed about our progress in helping animals through our newsletters and action alerts. For more information about NAVS, please turn to page 189.

Charitable giving and estate planning represent a profound personal decision of generosity. The listing of the charities below does not represent an endorsement by NAVS of any particular organization. This list, compiled by PCRM, simply provides you with specific information on one aspect of a charity's programming to assist you in making an informed decision. We encourage individuals to contact the charities themselves and to obtain additional information from the Council of Better Business Bureaus, Inc. at (703)276-0100 or the National Charities Information Bureau at (212)929-6300.

Health-Based Charities that DO NOT Fund Animal Research*

American Fund for Alternatives
to Animal Research
175 W. 12th St., Ste. 16G
New York, NY 10011

American Kidney Fund
6110 Executive Blvd., Ste. 1010
Rockville, MD 20852

American Leprosy Missions
1 ALM Way
Greenville, SC 29601

American Spinal Research Foundation
900 E. Tasman Dr.
San Jose, CA 95134

American Vitiligo Research Foundation
Box 7540
Clearwater, FL 34618

AmVets National Service Foundation
4647 Forbes Blvd.
Lanham, MD 20706

Arthritis Research Institute of America
300 S. Duncan Ave., Ste. 240
Clearwater, FL 34615

Association of Birth Defect Children
930 Woodcock Rd., Ste. 225
Orlando, FL 32803

Better Hearing Institute
P.O. Box 1840
Washington, DC 20013

The Cancer Project
5100 Wisconsin Ave., NW
Suite 404
Washington, DC 20016

* *Courtesy of Physicians Committee for Responsible Medicine, 5100 Wisconsin Ave., Suite 404, Washington, D.C. 20016, Phone: (202)686-2210.*

Child Health Foundation
10630 Little Patuxent Parkway
Century Plaza, Ste. 325
Columbia, MD 21044

Children's Burn Foundation
4929 Van Nuys Blvd.
Sherman Oaks, CA 91403

Children's Diagnostic Center, Inc.
2100 Pleasant Ave.
Hamilton, OH 45015

Children's Immune Disorder
16888 Greenfield Rd.
Detroit, MI 48221

Children's Organ Transplant
Fund of America
P.O. Box 650
Hendersonville, TN 37077

Design Industries
Foundation for AIDS
150 W. 26th St., Ste. 602
New York, NY 10001

Disability Rights Education &
Defense Fund
2212 Sixth St.
Berkeley, CA 94710

Disabled American Veterans
P.O. Box 14301
Cincinnati, OH 45250-0301

Easter Seals
230 W. Monroe St., Suite 1800
Chicago, IL 60606-4703

Endometriosis Association
8585 N. 76th Place
Milwaukee, WI 53223

Foundation for the Junior Blind
5300 Angeles Vista Blvd.
Los Angeles, CA 90043

Heimlich Institute
Deaconess Hospital
311 Straight St.
Cincinnati, OH 45219

Help Hospitalized Veterans
2065 Kurtz St.
San Diego, CA 92110

International Eye Foundation
7801 Norfolk Ave., Ste. 200
Bethesda, MD 20814

International Foundation for
Functional Gastrointestinal Disorders
P.O. Box 17864
Milwaukee, WI 53217

League for the Hard of Hearing
71 W. 23rd St.
New York, NY 10010-4162

Little People's Research Fund, Inc.
80 Sister Pierre Dr.
Towson, MD 21204

MCS Referral and Resources
508 Westgate Rd.
Baltimore, MD 21229-2343

Multiple Sclerosis Association of
America
706 Haddonfield Rd.
Cherry Hill, NJ 08002

National Alliance of Breast Cancer
Organizations (NABCO)
9 E. 37th St., 10th Fl.
New York, NY 10016

National Assn. for the Craniofacially
Handicapped (FACES)
P.O. Box 11082
Chattanooga, TN 37401

National Federation of the Blind
1800 Johnson St., Ste. 300
Baltimore, MD 21230-4998

Preventive Medicine Research Institute
900 Bridgeway, Suite One
Sausalito, CA 94965

Puerto Rico Community Network
for Clinical Research on AIDS
One Stop Station, #30
P.O. Box 70292
San Juan, PR 00936

Rhumatoid Disease Foundation
(aka The Arthritis Fund)
7111 Sweetgum Dr., S.W., #A
Fairview, TN 37062-9384

Skin Cancer Foundation
245 Fifth Ave., Suite 1403
New York, NY 10016

Spinal Cord Injury Network Int'l
3911 Princeton Dr.
Santa Rosa, CA 95405

The Thyroid Society
7515 South Main St.
Suite 545
Houston, TX 77030

Trauma Foundation
Mary Martin Trauma Center
San Francisco General Hospital
Building One, Room 300
1001 Potrero Ave.
San Francisco, CA 94110

United Amputee Services
P.O. Box 4277
Winter Park, FL 32793

United Cancer Research Society
3545 20th St.
Highland, CA 92346-4542

Vulvar Pain Foundation
P.O. Drawer 177
Graham, NC 27253

Health-Based Charities that STILL Fund Animal Research*

Alzheimer's Association
(aka Alzheimer's Disease and Related
Disorders Association)
919 N. Michigan Ave., Ste. 1000
Chicago, IL 60611-1676

Alzheimer's Disease Research
15825 Shady Grove Road, Ste. 140
Rockville, MD 20850

American Cancer Society
1599 Clifton Road, N.E.
Atlanta, GA 30329

American Diabetes Association
1660 Duke St.
Alexandria, VA 22314

American Federation for
Aging Research
1414 Ave. of the Americas, 18th Fl.
New York, NY 10019

American Foundation for
AIDS Research
120 Wall St., 13th Fl.
New York, NY 10005

American Heart Association
7272 Greenville Ave.
Dallas, TX 75321-4596

American Institute for Cancer Research
1759 R. St., N.W.
Washington, DC 20009

American Lung Association
National Headquarters
1740 Broadway
New York, NY 10019

American Paralysis Foundation
500 Morris Ave.
Springfield, NJ 07081

American Parkinson Disease Assn.
1250 Hylan Blvd.
Staten Island, NY 10305

American Red Cross
430 17th St., N.W.
Washington, DC 20006

American Tinnitus Association
P.O. Box 5
Portland, OR 97207-0005

Courtesy of Physicians Committee for Responsible Medicine, 5100 Wisconsin Ave., Suite 404, Washington, D.C. 20016, Phone: (202)686-2210.

Amyotrophic Lateral Sclerosis Assn.
21021 Ventura Blvd., Ste. 321
Woodland Hills, CA 91364

Arthritis Foundation
1330 W. Peachtree St.
Atlanta, GA 30309

Boys Town National Research
Hospital
555 N. 30th St.
Omaha, NE 68131

Canadian Diabetes Association
102-310 Broadway
Winnipeg, MB, R3C OS6 Canada

Cancer Research Foundation of
America
1600 Duke St., Ste. 110
Alexandria, VA 22314-3421

Christopher Reeve Foundation
P.O. Box 277, FDR Station
New York, NY 10150-0277

City of Hope
208 W. 8th St.
Los Angeles, CA 90014

Coronary Heart Disease Research
(program of the American Health
Assistance Foundation)
15825 Shady Grove Rd., Ste. 140
Rockville, MD 20850

Cystic Fibrosis Foundation
6931 Arlington Road
Bethesda, MD 20814

Deafness Research Foundation
575 5th Ave., 11th Fl.
New York, NY 10017

Eastern Paralyzed Veterans Association
7 Mill Brook Road
Wilton, NH 03086

Elizabeth Glazer Pediatric AIDS
Foundation
1311 Colorado Ave.
Santa Monica, CA 90404

Epilepsy Foundation of America
4351 Garden City Dr., Ste. 500
Landover, MD 20785

Families of Spinal Muscular Atrophy
P.O. Box 196
Libertyville, IL 60048-0196

The Foundation Fighting Blindness
(formerly National Retinitis
Pigmentosa Foundation)
Executive Plaza One
11350 McCormick Rd. Ste. 800
Hunt Valley, MD 21031-1014

Heart and Stroke Foundation of
Manitoba
352 Donald St., Ste. 301
Winnipeg, MB, R3B 2H8 Canada

Huntington's Disease
Society of America
744 Dulaney Valley Rd.
Towson, MD 21204

Joslin Diabetes Center
One Joslin Pl.
Boston, MA 02215

Juvenile Diabetes Foundation Int'l
120 Wall St.
New York, NY 10005-4001

Leukemia Society of America
600 3rd Ave.
New York, NY 10016

March of Dimes Birth Defects
Foundation
1275 Mamaroneck Ave.
White Plains, NY 10605

Massachusetts Lions Eye Research Fund
(Lions Club International Foundation)
118 Allen St.
Hampden, MA 01036

Memorial Sloan-Kettering
Cancer Center
1275 York Ave.
New York, NY 10021

The Miami Project to Cure Paralysis
P.O. Box 016960, R-48
Miami, FL 33101

Muscular Dystrophy Association
3300 E. Sunrise Dr.
Tucson, AZ 85718-3208

National Alliance for Research of
Schizophrenia and Depression
60 Cutter Mill Rd., Suite 200
Great Neck, NY 11021

National Alliance for the Mentally Ill
200 N. Glebe Rd., Suite 1015
Arlington, VA 22203-3754

National Foundation for Cancer Research
7315 Wisconsin Ave., Ste. 500 W.
Bethesda, MD 20814

National Headache Foundation
428 W. St. James Place, 2nd Fl.
Chicago, IL 60614-2750

National Hemophilia Foundation
116 West 32nd St., 11th Fl.
New York, NY 10001

National Kidney Foundation
30 E. 33rd St.
New York, NY 10016

National Multiple Sclerosis Society
733 3rd Ave., 6th Floor
New York, NY 10017-3288

National Osteoporosis Foundation
1150 17th St., N.W., Suite 500
Washington, DC 20036

National Parkinson Foundation
1501 N.W. 9th Ave.
Miami, FL 33136

National Psoriasis Foundation
6600 S.W. 92nd Ave., Ste. 300
Portland, OR 97223-7195

National Stroke Association
96 Inverness Dr. E, Suite I
Englewood, CO 80112-5112

National Vitiligo Foundation, Inc.
P.O. Box 6337
Tyler, TX 75711

Nina Hyde Center for
Breast Cancer Research
Lombardi Cancer Research Ctr.
3800 Reservoir Road, N.W.
Washington, DC 20007

Paralyzed Veterans of America
801 18th St., N.W.
Washington, DC 20006-3715

Parkinson's Disease Foundation
710 W. 168th St.
New York, NY 10032-9982

Research to Prevent Blindness
645 Madison Ave., 21st Fl.
New York, NY 10022-1010

St. Jude's Children's Research Hospital
501 St. Jude Place
Memphis, TN 38105

Shriners Hospitals for Children
2900 Rocky Point Dr.
Tampa, FL 33607

Susan G. Komen Breast
Cancer Foundation
5005 LBJ Freeway, Suite 370
Dallas, TX 75244

Tourette Syndrome Association
42-40 Bell Blvd.
Bayside, NY 11361-2820

United Cerebral Palsy
1660 L. St., N.W., Ste. 700
Washington, DC 20036

United Parkinson Foundation
833 W. Washington Blvd.
Chicago, IL 60607

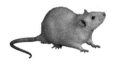

Ingredients Derived From Animals*

The following is a list of products containing animal-derived ingredients.

In addition to avoiding products that are animal tested, many individuals are committed to eliminating products which contain animal by-products. However, determining whether an ingredient listed on a product label comes from a plant, animal or synthetic process can be difficult, since many of the terms are not familiar to the average consumer. Complicating matters, many ingredients can come from more than one source—plant, animal or synthetically derived—and it is often impossible to tell from the label which source is being used.

To help clarify the origin of typical ingredients used in the manufacture of food, clothing, cosmetics, personal care and household products, we have provided the following lists of ingredients that are *always* derived from animals and those that *may be* derived from animals.

Ingredients which are *always* animal derived:

Albumin	Anchovy	Aspic
Aliphatic Alcohol	Angora	Astrakhan
Ambergris	Animal Oils and	Bee Products
Amniotic Fluid	Fats	Bee Pollen
Amylase	Arachidonic Acid	Beeswax

*From the American Vegan Society's "Listing of Ingredients and Materials: Animal, Vegetable or Mineral?" Reprinted with permission. For a complete listing (which includes definitions), contact the American Vegan Society at 56 Dinshah Drive, P.O. Box H, Malaga, NJ 08328. Tel. (609) 694-2887.

Bone Ash
Bone Meal
Bonito Flakes
Brawn
Carmine/
  Carminic Acid
Casein
Cashmere
Castoreum (Castor)
  (Do not confuse with
  Castor Oil, which is
  derived from the castor
  bean.)
Catgut
Caviar
Chamois
Chitin
Cholesterin, Choles-
  terol
Chole-Calciferol
Civit
Cochineal
Cod Liver Oil
Coral
Cortico Steroid
Down
Duodenum Substances
Egg Albumin
Egg Protein

Egg White
Eider Down
Elastin
Enzymes
Feathers
Felt
Fish Liver Oil
Fish Scales
Fur
Gelatin
Glycerides
Guanine
Hide
Hide Glue
Honey
Horsehair
Isinglass
Lactose
Lanolin (also,
  Lanol or Lanate
  derivatives)
Lard
Leather
Lipase
Luna Sponge
Milk Protein
Mink Oil
Mohair
Musk

Oleoic Oil
Oleostearin
Parchment
Pearl
Pearl, Cultured
Pepsin
Placenta
Polypeptides
Progesterone
Propolis
Quaternium 27
RNA/DNA
Roe
Royal Jelly
Sable
Shellac
Silk
Sodium 5'-Inosinate
Sperm Oil
Spermaceti Wax
Squalene/Squalane
Suede
Suet
Tallow
Testosterone
Vellum
Vitamin D3
Whey
Wool

The following ingredients *may be* derived from an animal, plant or synthetic source. You may have to contact the manufacturer to find out for certain whether an ingredient used in a particular product is derived from animals:

Adrenaline
Allantoin
Amino Acids
Anticaking Agent
Aspartic Acid
Bristle
Calcium Stearate
Caprylic Acid
Carmel
Cetyl Alcohol
Charcoal
Clarifying Agent
Collagen
Coloring
Cortisone
Cysteine L-Form,
   Cystine
Deoxy-ribonucleic acid
Emulsifiers
Estrogen
Fatty Acids

Flavorings
Gelling Agent
Glazing Agent
Glutamic Acid
Glycerin
Humectants
Hydrolized
   Proteins
Insulin
Keratin
L'Cysteine
   Hydrochloride
Lactic Acid
Lecithin
Linoleic Acid
Lipoids/Lipids
Lutein
Magnesium
   Stearate
Maple Sugar
Natural Source

Nucleic Acid
Nutrients
Octyl Dodecanol
Oleic Acid
Palmitic Acid
Panthenol
Polypeptides
Proteases
Releasing Agents
Rennet
Ribonucleic Acid
Solvent
Sponge
Stabilizers
Stearates/Stearic Acid
Steroid
Sugar
Urea
Velvet
Vitamin A
Vitamin B12

List of Responding Companies That DO and DO NOT Test on Animals

Here is a guide to the symbols used in this section. This information also appears on the back cover flap. Use this flap as a convenient reference as you look for your favorite products.

❤ This company is cruelty free. It DOES NOT test products or ingredients on animals, nor do any of its outside suppliers.

❥ This individual subsidiary/division DOES NOT test its products or ingredients on animals even though its parent company DOES test on animals.

◆ While this company DOES NOT test its *finished* products or ingredients on animals, it has no agreement with its suppliers stating that they do not test their *ingredients* on animals.

▼ This company DOES test products and/or ingredients on animals.

Additional symbols used after each company name:
❋ Company does not use any animal-derived ingredients in its products.
■ Company is a *manufacturer.*
● Company is a *distributor.*
▣ Company is a *mail-order company.*

◆ A-1 Bleach
(see James Austin Co.)

❤ 20 Mule Team Borax
(see Dial Corporation)

❤ 252 Spray
(see Ancient Formulas Inc.)

▼ 3M™ ■
Building 225-3S-05
St. Paul, MN 55144-1000
(800)3M-494-3M, (651)733-1110
Household

▼ 3M™ Dirtstop™ Mats
(see 3M™)

▼ 3M™ Trizact Abrasives
(see 3M™)

▼ A&M Products ■
83 Wooster Heights Rd.
Danbury, CT 06810
(203)731-2300
(see parent Clorox Company)
Companion animal

◆ A.J. Funk & Co. ✳ ■
1471 Timber Dr.
Elgin, IL 60123
(847)741-6760
Household

❤ ABBA Pure & Natural
Hair Care ✳ ■ ●
7400 E. Tierra Buena Ln.
Scottsdale, AZ 85260
(800)848-4475
(see parent Styling Technology Corp.)
Personal care

◆ ABCO, Inc. ■
2450 S. Watney Way #2519
Fairfield, CA 94533-6730
(800)678-2226
Personal care

❤ ABEnterprises ✳ ✉
247 W. 38th St.
New York, NY 10018
(212)997-2307
Personal care, Household

❤ Abkit, Inc. ■
207 East 94th St., 2nd Fl.
New York, NY 10128
(800)CAMOCARE, (212)860-8358
Personal care

❤ Abra Therapeutics ✳ ■
10365 Highway 116
Forestville, CA 95436
(707)869-0761
Personal care

❤ Absolute Aloe, Int'l. ✳ ■
P.O. Box 262
San Marcos, CA 92079-0262
(619)744-4483
Personal care, Cosmetics

▼ Act Fluoride Rinse
(see Johnson & Johnson)

❤ Adorisse Fragrance
(see Jafra Cosmetics Int'l)

- Adra Natural Soap ✳ ◼
  7955 Silverton Ave., Ste. 1201
  San Diego, CA 92126-6343
  (800)984-7627
  Personal care

- Adrien Arpel ✳ ● ⊠
  307 Treeworth Blvd.
  Broadview Heights, OH 44147
  (440)717-0860
  Personal care, Cosmetics

- Advanced Research Labs ◼
  151 Kalmus Dr., Ste. H-3
  Costa Mesa, CA 92626
  (800)966-6960
  Personal care

- Advanced Time Protector®
  Daily Defense Cream
  (see Jafra Cosmetics Int'l)

- ADWE Laboratories ✳ ◼ ●
  141 20th St.
  Brooklyn, NY 11232
  (718)788-6838
  Personal care, Cosmetics, Household

- African Pride
  (see Revlon, Inc.)

- ◆ African Royale
  (see Bronner Brothers)

- Age Defying Makeup
  (see Revlon, Inc.)

- Ageless Beauty
  (see Arizona Natural Resources, Inc.)

- Agree
  (see Schwarzkopf & Dep Inc.)

- Ahimsa Natural Beauty ✳ ◼ ●
  1250 Reid St., #13A
  Richmond Hill, Ontario
  L4B 1G3, Canada
  (905)709-8977
  Personal care

- ▼ Aim
  (see Chesebrough-Pond's USA Co.)

- Air Scense
  (see Shadow Lake, Inc.)

- Air Therapy®
  (see Mia Rose Products)

- ◆ Air-Scent
  (see Surco Products, Inc.)

- Aiyana Skin Care System
  (see Oxyfresh Worldwide, Inc.)

- ▼ Ajax
  (see Colgate-Palmolive Co.)

◆ AKA Saunders, Inc. ■ ●
1011 Gilman St.
Berkeley, CA 94710
(510)558-7100
Personal care

❤ Alaska Herb & Tea Co. ✳ ■ ● ⊠
6710 Weimer Dr.
Anchorage, AK 99502
(907)245-3499
Personal care

❤ Alba Botanica
(see Avalon Natural Products)

▼ Alberto-Culver Co. ■
2525 Armitage Ave.
Melrose Park, IL 60160
(708)450-3000
Personal care, Household

❤ Alexandra Avery Purely Natural
Body Care ■ ⊠
4717 SE Belmont
Portland, OR 97215
(800)669-1863, (503)236-5926
Personal care

▼ All Detergent
(see Lever Brothers)

◆ All Terrain Co. ✳ ■
315 1st St., Ste. U-274
Encinitas, CA 92024-3528
(800)246-7328
Personal care

❤ Allens Naturally ✳ ■ ⊠
P.O. Box 514, Dept. T
Farmington, MI 48332
(800)352-8971, (313)453-5410
Household

◆ Allergy Resources ✳ ■ ● ⊠
557 Burbank St., Ste. K
Broomfield, CO 80020
303-438-0600
*Personal care, Cosmetics,
Household, Companion animal*

❤ Allerpet, Inc. ✳ ■
P.O. Box 2220, Lenox Hill Station
New York, NY 10021
(212)861-1134
Companion animal

❤ Allon Personal Care Corp. ■ ● ⊠
25655 Springbrook Ave., #6
Saugus, CA 91350
(661)253-2723
Personal care

♥ Almay, Inc. ■ ●
625 Madison Ave.
New York, NY 10022
(see parent Revlon, Inc.)
Cosmetics

♥ Aloe Commodities Inc. ■
2161 Hutton Dr., Ste. 126
Carrollton, TX 75006-0333
(972)241-4251
Personal care

♥ Aloe Complete ✳ ■
P.O.Box 67
Vista, CA 92085-0067
(800)464-2563, (619)279-0727
Personal care, Cosmetics

♥ Aloe Creme Laboratories ■ ● ▣
335 New Road
Monmouth Junction, NJ 08852
(800)327-4969, (732)438-8998
Personal care, Cosmetics

◆ Aloe Oat Bath
(see Espree Animal Products)

♥ Aloe Vera Freeze Dried Powder
(see Absolute Aloe, Int'l)

♥ Aloegen
(see Levlad, Inc.)

◆ Aloette Cosmetics, Inc. ●
4900 Highlands Pkwy. SE
Smyrna, GA 30082-5132
(800)ALOETTE, (770)956-9700
Personal care, Cosmetics

♥ Alvera
(see Texas Best UnLimited, LP)

♥ Alvin Last, Inc. ✳ ■
425 Saw Mill River Rd.
Ardsley, NY 10502
(800)527-8123, (914)479-0900
Personal care

▼ Always
(see Procter & Gamble)

♥ AM Cosmetics, Inc. ■ ●
100 Porete Ave.
North Arlington, NJ 07031
(201)998-8890
Cosmetics

♥ Amazon Premium Products ✳ ■ ● ▣
275 NE 59th St.
Miami, FL 33137
(800)832-5645
*Personal care, Cosmetics,
Household, Companion animal*

◆ Amazon Rainflowers Herbal
Hair Care
(see Tropical Botanicals)

♥ Amberwood ✳ ✉
Route 2, Box 300, Baker County
Leary, GA 31762
(912)792-6246
*Personal care, Cosmetics,
Household, Companion animal*

♥ American Eco-Systems ✳ ■ ●
125 9th St., P.O. Box 109
Wellman, IA 52356
(319)646-2943
Household

♥ American Formulating & Mfg. ✳ ■
350 West Ash St., #700
San Diego, CA 92101
(714)781-6860
Personal care, Household

♥ American Int'l Ind. ■
2220 Gaspar Ave.
Los Angeles, CA 90040
(800)621-9585, (323)728-4464
Personal care, Cosmetics

♥ American Safety Razor Co. ■
One Razor Blade Lane
Verona, VA 24482-0979
(800)445-9284, (540)248-8000
Personal care

◆ America's Finest Products Corp. ✳ ■
1639 9th St.
Santa Monica, CA 90404
(310)450-6555
Household

◆ Amla Conditioner
(see ShiKai Products)

◆ Amon-Re Laboratories ✳ ■
210 Commercial Dr.
Thomasville, GA 31757
(912)228-1284
Personal care

◆ Amoresse Laboratories ■
3435 Wilshire Blvd., Ste. 975
Los Angeles, CA 90010-1998
(800)258-7931
Cosmetics

♥ Amrita Aromatherapy, Inc. ■ ●
1900 W. Stone Ave.
Fairfield, IA 52556-2152
(515)472-9136
Personal care, Cosmetics

◆ Amway Corp. ■
7575 Fulton St. East
Ada, MI 49355-0001
(616)787-6000
Personal care, Cosmetics, Household

◆ Anais Anais
(see L'Oreal of Paris)

♥ Ancient Formulas Inc. ■ ●
638 W. 33rd St. North
Wichita, KS 67204
(800)543-3026, (316)838-5600
Personal care

♥ Anew
(see Avon Products, Inc.)

◆ Angel Soft Bath Tissue
(see Georgia-Pacific Corp.)

◆ Animale Parfums
(see Parlux Fragrances, Inc.)

♥ Annemarie Borlind
(see Borlind of Germany)

♥ Anthe-Essence Aromatherapy ✳ ■
P.O. Box 891342
Temecula, CA 92589-1342
(909)677-4412
Personal care, Companion animal

◆ Anthony G. Therapeutic Pet Products
(see Carina Supply Inc.)

♥ Aphrodisia Naturals
(see Aphrodisia Products, Inc.)

♥ Aphrodisia Products, Inc. ■ ● ✉
62 Kent St.
Brooklyn, NY 11222
(718)383-3677
Personal care

♥ Apiana
(see Baudelaire, Inc.)

♥ Appleberry Attic ■ ✉
P.O. Box 135361
Clermont, FL 34713-5361
(800)633-2682
Personal care, Companion animal

◆ Aqua Di Gio
(see L'Oreal of Paris)

▼ Aqua Net
(see Chesebrough-Pond's USA Co.)

▼ Aquafresh
(see SmithKline Beecham
Consumer Healthcare)

♥ Arabella Stuart
(see Cosmetique, Inc.)

♥ Aramis
(see Estee Lauder Companies)

♥ Arbico Environmentals ✳ ■ ● ▨
P.O. Box 4247
Tucson, AZ 85738-1247
(520)825-9785
*Personal care, Cosmetics,
Household, Companion animal*

◆ Arbonne Int'l ✳ ●
15 Argonaut
Aliso Viejo, CA 92656
(800)ARBONNE, (949)770-2610
Personal care, Cosmetics

♥ Ardell Int'l Inc. ■
2220 Gaspar Ave.
City of Industry, CA 90040
(323)728-2999
(see parent American Int'l Ind.)
Personal care, Cosmetics

♥ Arizona Natural Resources ■
2525 E. Beardsley Rd.
Phoenix, AZ 85024
(602)569-6900
Personal care, Cosmetics

♥ Arizona Naturals Desert Botanicals
(see Arizona Natural Resources, Inc.)

▼ Arm & Hammer
(see Church & Dwight Co., Inc.)

▼ Armor All Products Group ■
1221 Broadway St.
Oakland, CA 94612
(510)271-7000
(see parent Clorox Company)
Household

▼ Armstrong Floor Cleaners
(see S.C. Johnson & Son, Inc.)

♥ Aroma Life Co. ✳ ■
P.O. Box 7371
Van Nuys, CA 91409
(805)944-4909
Personal care, Cosmetics

◆ Aroma Medica ■
900 Bethlehem Pike
Glenside, PA 19038
(215)233-5210
Personal care, Cosmetics

♥ Aroma Terra ✳ ■ ● ▨
P.O. Box 83027
Phoenix, AZ 83071-3027
(800)456-3765, (602)371-4676
Personal care

♥ Aroma Vera, Inc. ✳ ■ ●
5901 Rodeo Rd.
Los Angeles, CA 90016
(800)669-9514
Personal care

❤ Aromaland, Inc. ■ ●
1326 Rufina Circle
Santa Fe, NM 87505
(800)933-5267, (505)438-0402
Personal care, Household

❤ Aromascape
(see Jafra Cosmetics Int'l)

❤ AromaTherapeutix ✱ ▣
P.O. Box 2908
Seal Branch, CA 90740
(800)308-6284
Personal care

❤ Aromatic Relief
(see East End Imports, Co.)

◆ ARTec Systems Group Inc. ✱ ■
99 Seaview Blvd.
Port Washington, NY 11050
(516)625-6663
Personal care

◆ Artistry® Skin Care & Cosmetics
(see Amway Corp.)

❤ Artmatic Cosmetics
(see AM Cosmetics, Inc.)

❤ Atra
(see Gillette Co.)

❤ Attar Bazaar
(see Chishti Co.)

▼ Attends
(see Procter & Gamble)

❤ Aubrey Organics ■
4419 N. Manhattan Ave.
Tampa, FL 33614
(800)282-7394, (813)877-4186
*Personal care, Cosmetics,
Household, Companion animal*

❤ Auroma Int'l, Inc. ■
P.O. Box 1008
Silver Lake, WI 53170
(262)889-8569
Personal care, Cosmetics

❤ Auromere Ayurvedic Imports ▣
2621 West Hwy. 12
Lodi, CA 95242
(800)735-4691, (209)339-3710
Personal care, Cosmetics

◆ Aurora Henna Co. ■ ●
1507 E. Franklin Ave.
Minneapolis, MN 55404
(612)870-4456
Personal care

◆ Aurore Botanicals ✉
10767 Rose Ave., Apt. 28
Los Angeles, CA 90034-4423
(310)859-2232
Personal care

♥ Auroshikha
(see Auroma Int'l)

▶ Aussie Hair Care Products
(see Redmond Products, Inc.)

◆ Austin Carpet Cleaner
(see James Austin Co.)

◆ Austin Laundry Detergent
(see James Austin Co.)

♥ Austin-Rose® Inc.
(see Mia Rose Products)

◆ Automation, Inc. ✳ ■
11737 Central Pkwy.
Jacksonville, FL 32224
(800)617-4220, (904)998-9888
Household

♥ Avalon Natural Products ■ ● ✉
P.O. Box 750428
Petaluma, CA 94975-0428
(707)769-5120
Personal care, Cosmetics

♥ Avalon Organic Botanicals
(see Avalon Natural Products)

♥ Aveda Corporation ■
4000 Pheasant Ridge Dr.
Minneapolis, MN 55449
(800)AVEDA-24
(see parent Estee Lauder Companies)
Personal care, Cosmetics

▼ Aveeno
(see Johnson & Johnson)

▼ Aviance Fragrances
(see Chesebrough-Pond's USA Co.)

♥ Avon Products, Inc. ■ ●
1345 Ave. of the Americas
New York, NY 10105-0196
(800)367-2866, (212)282-5000
Personal care, Cosmetics

◆ Aware Diaper, Inc. ✳ ■
P.O. Box 2591
Greeley, CO 80632
(970)352-6822
Personal care

♥ Ayurveda Holistic Center ✳ ■ ● ✉
82A Bayville Ave.
Bayville, NY 11709
(516)628-8200
Companion animal

♥ Azida, Inc. ✳ ■ ⊠
P.O. Box 247
Elfrida, AZ 85610
(800)603-6601
Personal care

▼ Aziza Cosmetics
(see Chesebrough-Pond's USA Co.)

♥ Aztec Secret ✳ ■
P.O. Box 841
Pahrump, NV 89041-0841
(775)727-1882
Personal care

◆ Azur Fragrances USA, Inc. ✳ ●
50 East 42nd St., Ste. 2105
New York, NY 10017
(212)687-5566
Personal care

◆ Babaìu Body Lotion
(see Tropical Botanicals)

▼ Babe
(see Chesebrough-Pond's USA Co.)

▼ Baby Bath
(see Mennen Co.)

▼ Baby Magic
(see Mennen Co.)

◆ Baby Orajel
(see Del Laboratories, Inc.)

♥ Baby Touch
(see Studio Magic)

♥ Back to Basics
(see Smith & Vandiver)

♥ Back to Nature, Inc. ✳ ● ⊠
5627 N. Milwaukee Ave.
Chicago, IL 60646
(773)583-0402
*Personal care, Cosmetics,
Household, Companion animal*

♥ BacOut™ Stain & Odor
Eliminator
(see Bio-O-Kleen Industries, Inc.)

♥ Bain de Beaute
(see Arizona Natural Resources, Inc.)

▼ Bain de Soleil
(see Procter & Gamble)

▼ Balm Barr
(see Mennen Co.)

▼ Balmex® Diaper Rash Ointment
(see Black Drug Co.)

▼ Banana Boat
(see Playtex Products, Inc.)

❤ Banana Republic M Fragrance
(see Gap, Inc.)

❤ Banana Republic W Fragrance
(see Gap, Inc.)

❤ Banana Republic Classic Fragrance
(see Gap, Inc.)

❤ Banana Republic Modern Fragrance
(see Gap, Inc.)

▼ Band-Aid
(see Johnson & Johnson)

▼ Banner
(see Procter & Gamble)

◆ Bar Keepers Friend
(see SerVaas Laboratories Inc.)

❤ Bare Escentuals ■ ● ⊠
600 Townsend St., Ste. 329 East
San Francisco, CA 94103
(800)227-3990, (415)487-3400
Personal care, Cosmetics

❤ Bare Foot
(see Dial Corporation)

◆ Baryshnikov Parfums
(see Parlux Fragrances, Inc.)

◆ Basch Co., Inc. ✳ ■
P.O. Box 188
Freeport, NY 11520
(516)378-8100
Household

❤ Basically Natural ✳ ⊠
109 East G St.
Brunswick, MD 21716
(800)352-7099, (301)834-7923
*Personal care, Cosmetics,
Household, Companion animal*

❤ Bath & Body Works ✳ ■
7 Limited Pkwy.
Reynoldsburg, OH 43068
(800)395-1001, (614)856-6310
(see parent Limited, Inc.)
*Personal care, Cosmetics,
Household*

❤ Bath Island, Inc. ■
469 Amsterdam Ave.
New York, NY 10024
(212)787-9415
*Personal care, Household,
Companion animal*

❤ Baudelaire, Inc. ●
166 Emerald St.
Keene, NH 03431
(800)327-2324, (603)352-9234
Personal care

▼ Bausch & Lomb Inc. ■
One Bausch & Lomb Pl.
Rochester, NY 14604
(800)344-8815, (716)338-6000
Personal care

❤ Bavarian Alpenol & Sunspirit ✳ ■
1343 N. Nevada Ave.
Colorado Springs, CO 80903
(719)633-8931
Personal care

❤ Baxter Environmental Products,
Inc. DBA Nala Berry Labs ✳ ■
P.O. Box 151
Palm Desert, CA 92261
(760)568-9446
Companion animal

◆ Beaumont Products, Inc. ✳ ■
1560 Big Shanty Rd.
Kennesaw, GA 30144
(800)451-7096, (770)514-9000
*Personal care, Household,
Companion animal*

❤ Beautiful
(see Estee Lauder Companies)

❤ Beauty For All Seasons, Inc. ●
P.O. Box 51810, 360 B St.
Idaho Falls, ID 83405-1810
(800)942-4336, (208)525-7800
Personal care, Cosmetics

❤ Beauty Naturally, Inc. ■ ▣
P.O. Box 4905
Burlingame, CA 94010
(650)697-1809
Personal care

❤ Beauty Without Cruelty Cosmetics
(see Avalon Natural Products)

❤ Bebe
(see Baudelaire, Inc.)

❤ Beehive Botanicals Inc. ■ ▣
Box 8257
Hayward, WI 54843
(800)283-4274, (715)634-4274
Personal care

❤ Belle Star, Inc. ■ ▣
23151 Alcalde Dr., Ste. A-1
Laguna Hills, CA 92653-1419
(949)768-7006
Personal care

▼ Ben Nye Makeup ▪
5935 Bowcroft St.
Los Angeles, CA 90016
(310)839-1984
Cosmetics

❤ Benetton USA Corp. ▪
597 Fifth Ave., 11th Fl.
New York, NY 10017
(800)535-4491, (305)594-6661
Personal care, Cosmetics

❤ Beta-Ginseng®
(see Earth Science, Inc.)

▼ Better Off
(see Playtex Products, Inc.)

▼ Beyond Time Facial Crème
(see Marche Image Corp.)

❤ Bill Blass, Inc. ▪
625 Madison Ave.
New York, NY 10022
(212)527-5000
(see parent Revlon, Inc.)
Cosmetics

▼ Binanca
(see Playtex Products, Inc.)

❤ Bio Pac Inc. ✳ ▪
584 Pinto Ct.
Incline Village, NV 89451
(800)225-2855
Personal care, Household

❤ Biogime Int'l, Inc. ✳ ▪ ● ⌨
25602 IH-45 North Fwy.
Spring, TX 77386
(800)338-8784, (281)298-2607
Personal care

❤ Bi-O-Kleen Industries, Inc. ✳ ▪
P.O. Box 82066
Portland, OR 97282-0066
(503)557-0216
Household

❥ Biolage
(see Matrix Essentials, Inc.)

❤ Biologica®
(see Earth Science, Inc.)

◆ BioMedic Clinical Care ▪ ⌨
4602 E. Hammond Lane
Phoenix, AZ 85034
(800)736-5155
Personal care, Cosmetics

◆ Bio-Organic Basic Shampoo
(see Espree Animal Products, Inc.)

❤ BioProgress Technology, Ltd. ✳ ■
Unit 1, Norwood Rd., March
Cambridgeshire, PE15 8QD
United Kingdom
(770)641-0264, (+44)1354-655-674
Personal care

❤ Bio-Skin Care
(see Beauty Naturally, Inc.)

▼ BioSun
(see Playtex Products)

◆ Biotherm Cosmetics & Skin Care
(see L'Oreal of Paris)

▼ Biz
(see Procter & Gamble)

▼ Black Flag
(see Clorox Company)

❤ Black Radiance Cosmetics
(see AM Cosmetics, Inc.)

❤ Blessed Herbs ▣
109 Barre Plains Rd.
Oakham, MA 01068
(508)882-3839
Personal care

◆ Blistex, Inc. ■
1800 Swift Dr.
Oak Brook, IL 60523
(630)571-2870
Personal care

▼ Block Drug Co. ■
257 Cornelison Ave.
Jersey City, NJ 07302
(201)434-3000
Personal care

❤ Blue 655 Fragrance
(see Gap, Inc.)

◆ Blue Cross Beauty Products, Inc. ✳■
12251 Montague St.
Pacoima, CA 91331
(818)896-8681
Cosmetics

▼ Blue Grass
(see Elizabeth Arden Co.)

❤ Blue Pearl
(see Siddha Int'l)

❤ Blue Ribbons Pet Care ✳ ▣
1442 Peters Blvd.
Bay Shore, NY 11706-3946
(800)552-BLUE
Companion animal

♥ Bob Kelly Cosmetics ■
151 West 46th St.
New York, NY 10036
(212)819-0030
Cosmetics

♥ Bobbi Brown Essentials
(see Estee Lauder Companies)

♥ Bocabelli Inc. ✳ ●
4004 Avondale Lane, NW
Canton, OH 44708-1618
(330)477-9048
Personal care

♥ Body & Soul Aromatherapy ✳ ■
2073 3rd St.
Livermore, CA 94550-4414
(925)443-8887
Personal care

♥ Body & Soul of Chicago ✉
212 N. Shore Dr.
Oakwood Hills, IL 60013
(800)272-7085
Personal care

♥ Body Crystal Environmental
Products ✳ ■
P.O. Box 331
Dana Point, CA 92629
(714)448-8832
*Personal care, Cosmetics,
Companion animal*

♥ Body Encounters ✳ ✉
604 Manor Rd.
Cinnaminson, NJ 08077
(800)839-2639, (856)829-4660
Personal care

◆ Body Guard Pet Food Supplement
(see Pro-Tec Pet Health)

◆ Body Satin
(see Granny's Old Fashioned
Products)

♥ Body Sense—
Midwest/BodeWell Ltd. ✳ ●
212 N. Shore Dr.
Oakwood Hills, IL 60013
(888)539-7018
Personal care

♥ Body Shop ■ ✉
5036 One World Way
Wake Forest, NC 27587
(919)554-4900
Personal care, Cosmetics

♥ Body Time ● ✉
1101 Eighth St., Ste. 100
Berkeley, CA 94710
(510)524-0216
Personal care

- ❤ Body Tools ■ ● ⬚
  16 Pamaron Way, Ste. C
  Novato, CA 94949-6217
  (415)382-1355
  Personal care

- ❤ BodyLind Products
  (see Borlind of Germany)

- ❤ Bodyography ■ ⬚
  1641 16th St.
  Santa Monica, CA 90404
  (310)399-2886
  Personal care, Cosmetics

- ▼ Bold
  (see Procter & Gamble)

- ▼ Bone Strait
  (see Alberto-Culver Co.)

- ❤ Bonne Bell, Inc. ■
  18519 Detroit Ave.
  Lakewood, OH 44107
  (800)321-1006, (216)221-0800
  Personal care, Cosmetics

- ▼ Bo-Peep
  (see Church & Dwight Co., Inc.)

- ◆ Borage
  (see ShiKai Products)

- ❤ Borateem® Bleach
  (see Dial Corporation)

- ❤ Boraxo® Soap
  (see Dial Corporation)

- ❤ Borghese Cosmetics
  (see Revlon, Inc.)

- ❤ Borlind of Germany ■
  P.O. Box 130
  New London, NH 03257
  (800)447-7024, (603)526-2076
  Personal care, Cosmetics

- ❤ Born Again
  (see Alvin Last, Inc.)

- ▼ Boston® Brand
  (see Bausch & Lomb Inc.)

- ❤ Botanical Benefits™
  (see Nature's Sunshine Products)

- ❤ Botanical Products, Inc. ■ ●
  34725 Bogart Dr.
  Springville, CA 93265
  (559)539-3432
  Personal care

- ◆ Botanical Therapeutic Hair &
  Skin Care
  (see Carina Supply Inc.)

51

❤ Botanicals
(see Smith & Vandiver)

◆ Botanics of California ❋ ■
P.O. Box 384
Ukiah, CA 95482-0384
(707)462-6141
Personal care

▼ Bounce
(see Procter & Gamble)

▼ Bounty
(see Procter & Gamble)

◆ BP's Pet Odor Eliminator
(see Beaumont Products, Inc.)

◆ Bradford Soap Works, Inc. ■
P.O. Box 1007
West Warwick, RI 02893
(401)821-2141
Personal care

❤ Braun
(see Gillette Co.)

❤ Breath-Eze
(see St. JON Laboratories)

❤ Breck® Products
(see Dial Corporation)

▼ Breeze
(see Lever Brothers)

❤ Breezy Balms Oak Away
(see Simmons Natural Bodycare)

▼ Brillo Pads
(see Church & Dwight Co., Inc.)

▼ Bristol-Myers Squibb Co. ■
345 Park Ave.
New York, NY 10154-0037
(203)357-5226
Personal care

▼ Brita (USA), Inc. ■
1221 Broadway St.
Oakland, CA 94612
(510)271-7000
(see parent Clorox Company)
Household

▼ Brite Floor Polish
(see S.C. Johnson & Son, Inc.)

◆ Bronner Brothers ■
600 Bronner Brothers Way
Atlanta, GA 30310
(404)696-4000
Personal care

◆ Bronze Wash
(see Aloette Cosmetics, Inc.)

♥ Brookside Soap Co. ✳.■
P.O. Box 55638
Seattle, WA 98155
(425)742-2265
Personal care, Companion animal

▼ Bruce Floor Care
(see Church & Dwight Co., Inc.)

▼ Brut Products
(see Chesebrough-Pond's USA Co.)

♥ Bufette Buffers
(see Delby System)

♥ Buff Naked
(see Flowery Beauty Products)

♥ Bug Off
(see Sunfeather Natural Soap Co.)

♥ Bulgar Skin Care
(see East End Imports, Co.)

♥ Bump Fighter®
(see American Safety Razor Co.)

♥ Burma Shave®
(see American Safety Razor Co.)

♥ Burt's Bees ■
8221A Brownleigh Dr.
Raleigh, NC 27612-7409
(919)510-8720
Personal care, Companion animal

◆ Buty-Wave Products Co., Inc. ■
7323 Beverly Blvd.
Los Angeles, CA 90036
(323)936-2191
Personal care

♥ C.E. Hinds ✳ ■ ● ▨
300 Wildwood Ave.
Woburn, MA 01801
(800)874-4788
Personal care, Cosmetics

♥ CA-Botana Int'l, Inc. ✳ ■
9365 Waples St.
San Diego, CA 92121
(800)872-2332
Personal care

▼ Cachet Fragrance
(see Chesebrough-Pond's USA Co.)

♥ Cactus Juice Products
(see Safe Solutions, Inc.)

♥ Cadette
(see Cosmetique, Inc.)

♥ California Baby Botanical
Skin Care ✳ ◼
217 S. Linden Dr.
Beverly Hills, CA 90212-3704
(310)277-6430
Personal care

♥ California Gold Products
(see J & J Jojoba/California
Gold Products)

♥ California Mango ✳ ◼
16632 Burke Lane
Huntington Beach, CA 92647
(714)375-2599
Personal care

▼ Calvin Klein Cosmetics Co. ✳ ◼
Trump Tower, 725 Fifth Ave.
New York, NY 10022-2519
(973)347-8889, (212)719-2600
(see parent Unilever United
States Inc.)
Personal care, Cosmetics

▼ Camay
(see Procter & Gamble)

♥ Cambria Soap Co.
(see Exotic Nature Body
Care Products)

▼ Cameo® Metal Polish
(see Church & Dwight Co., Inc.)

♥ CamoCare
(see Abkit, Inc.)

♥ Canada's All Natural
Soap, Inc. ◼ ● ▨
P.O. Box 64567
Unionville, Ontario, L3R 0M9,
Canada
(905)415-1540
Personal care, Companion animal

▼ Carefree Panty Shields
(see Johnson & Johnson)

▼ Caress
(see Lever Brothers)

♥ Caribbean Bay Rum
(see Body Crystal
Environmental Products)

◆ Caribe Body Lotion
(see Aloette Cosmetics, Inc.)

◆ Carina Supply Inc. ✳ ◼
464 Granville St.
Vancouver, BC, V6C 1V4
Canada
(800)663-0479, (604)687-3617
Personal care, Companion animal

● Carma Laboratories, Inc. ■
5801 West Airways Ave.
Franklin, WI 53132
(414)421-7707
Personal care

● Carmex Lip Balm
(see Carma Laboratories, Inc.)

● Carrington Parfums Ltd. ■
625 Madison Ave.
New York, NY 10022
(212)527-5000
(see parent Revlon, Inc.)
Cosmetics

▼ Cascade
(see Procter & Gamble)

▼ Cashmere Bouquet
(see Colgate-Palmolive Co.)

● Cat Poo
(see Sunfeather Natural Soap Co.)

● Catherine Atzen Laboratories ■ ● ⊠
1790 Hamilton Ave.
San Jose, CA 95125
(800)468-4362, (408)265-0121
Personal care, Cosmetics

◆ Cat's Pride Cat Litter
(see Oil-Dri Corporation of America)

◆ CCA Industries, Inc. ■
200 Murray Hill Pkwy.
East Rutherford, NJ 07073
(201)935-3232, (201)330-1400
Personal care

● CD&P Health Products, Inc. ■ ●
P.O. Box 53
Nutley, NJ 07110
(800)922-0164
Personal care

● Celebrity Cosmetics
(see Studio Magic)

● Celestial Body ■ ● ⊠
21298 Pleasant Hill Rd.
Boonville, MO 65233
(800)882-6858
Personal care

● Cellular Defense Products
(see La Prairie, Inc.)

● Cellular Treatment Products
(see La Prairie, Inc.)

● Centenary
(see Auroma Int'l)

◆ Champion Skin and Coat Conditioner
(see Trophy Animal Health Care)

♥ Chandrika Ayurvedic Soap
(see Auroma Int'l)

♥ Chanel, Inc. ■
9 W. 57th St.
New York, NY 10019
(212)688-5055
Personal care, Cosmetics

♥ Change of Face Cosmetics ✳ ▣
P.O. Box 592
Hobart, IN 46342
(800)865-1755, (219)947-4040
Personal care, Cosmetics

♥ Charles of the Ritz Group Ltd. ■
625 Madison Ave.
New York, NY 10022
(212)527-4000
(see parent Revlon, Inc.)
Personal care, Cosmetics

♥ Charlie
(see Revlon, Inc.)

▼ Charmin
(see Procter & Gamble)

▼ Cheer
(see Procter & Gamble)

◆ Chem Pro ✳ ■ ▣
P.O. Box 2708
Spartanburg, SC 29304-2708
(800)835-3712
Household

◆ Chempak Industries
(see Hi-Lex Corp.)

▼ Chesebrough-Pond's USA Co. ■
33 Benedict Pl.
Greenwich, CT 06830
(800)786-5135, (203)661-2000
(see parent Unilever United States Inc.)
Personal care

▼ Chimere
(see Prince Matchabelli)

♥ Chishti Co. ✳ ■
P.O. Box 7249
Endicott, NY 13761-7249
(800)344-7172, (607)748-2220
Personal care

▼ Chloe
(see Elizabeth Arden Co.)

▼ Chore Boy
(see Reckitt & Colman)

◆ Christine Valmy ■
285 Change Bridge Rd.
Pine Brook, NJ 07058
(800)526-5057, (201)575-1050
Personal care, Cosmetics

▼ Chubs
(see Playtex Products)

❤ Chuckles, Inc. ✳ ■ ●
P.O. Box 5126
Manchester, NH 03108-5126
(800)221-3496, (603)669-4228
Personal care

▼ Church & Dwight Co., Inc. ■
P.O. Box 1625
Horsham, PA 19044-6625
(800)524-1328, (609)683-5900
Household

❤ CiCi Cosmetics ●
215 N. Eucalyptus Ave.
Inglewood, CA 90301
(800)869-1224, (310)680-9696
Cosmetics

❤ Citra Science Horse Care Products
(see Vin-Dotco, Inc.)

❤ Citra-Glow®
(see Mia Rose Products)

❤ Citra-Solv
(see Shadow Lake, Inc.)

❤ Citre Shine
(see Advanced Research Labs)

◆ Citrus Magic Products
(see Beaumont Products, Inc.)

◆ Citrusil™
(see Espree Animal Products, Inc.)

▼ cK be
(see Calvin Klein Cosmetics Co.)

▼ cK one
(see Calvin Klein Cosmetics Co.)

❧ Clairol, Inc. ■
One Blachley Rd.
Stamford, CT 06922
(800)223-5800, (203)357-5200
(see parent Bristol-Myers Squibb Co.)
Personal care

❤ Clarins of Paris ✳ ■ ●
135 East 57th St., 15th Fl.
New York, NY 10022
(212)980-1800
Personal care, Cosmetics

▼ Clarion Cosmetics ■
11050 York Rd.
Hunt Valley, MD 21030
(410)785-7300
(see parent Procter & Gamble)
Cosmetics

❤ Classic Cosmetics, Inc. ✳ ■
9601 Irondale Ave.
Chatsworth, CA 91311
(818)773-9042
Personal care, Cosmetics

❤ Classic Fragrances Ltd. ✳ ●
26 W. 17th St.
New York, NY 10011
(212)929-2266, (212)371-6300
Cosmetics

▼ Clean & Clear
(see Johnson & Johnson)

◆ Clean Shower
(see Automation, Inc.)

❤ Clean Zyme
(see Beauty Naturally, Inc.)

❤ Clear Conscience, LLC ✳ ■ ✉
P.O. Box 17855
Arlington, VA 22216
(800)595-9592, (703)527-7566
Personal care

❤ Clear Light The Cedar
Company ■ ● ✉
Box 551—State Rd. 165
Placitas, NM 87043
(800)557-3463, (505)867-2381
Personal care, Cosmetics, Household

❤ Clear Spring
(see Faith Products Ltd.)

▼ Clearasil
(see Procter & Gamble)

❤ Clearly Natural Products ✳ ■
P.O. Box 750024
Petaluma, CA 94975-0024
(800)274-7627, (707)762-5815
Personal care

❤ Clearskin
(see Avon Products, Inc.)

❤ Clientele ■ ● ✉
14101 N.W. Fourth St.
Sunrise, FL 33325-6209
(954)845-9500
Personal care, Cosmetics

❤ Clinique Beauty Products
(see Estee Lauder Companies)

▼ Clorox Company ■
1221 Broadway
Oakland, CA 94612
(510)271-7000
Household, Companion animal

▼ Close-Up
(see Chesebrough-Pond's USA Co.)

▼ Coast
(see Procter & Gamble)

◆ Coat Guard Conditioning Shampoo
(see Pro-Tec Pet Health)

❤ Cold Wax Co. ✳ ■
P.O. Box 600476
San Diego, CA 92160
(619)283-0880
Personal care

▼ Colgate Instant Shave
(see Colgate-Palmolive Co.)

▼ Colgate Toothpastes
(see Colgate-Palmolive Co.)

▼ Colgate-Palmolive Co. ■
300 Park Ave.
New York, NY 10022-7499
(800)221-4607
Personal care, Household

❤ Colin Ingram Co. ✳ ■ ●
P.O. Box 146
Comptche, CA 95427-0146
(415)328-3184
Personal care

❤ Cologne Bouquet®
(see Hewitt Soap Co., Inc.)

◆ Colonial Dames Co. Ltd. ■
P.O. Box 22022
Los Angeles, CA 90022
(800)774-6441, (213)773-6441
Personal care

❤ Color Me Beautiful ●
14000 Thunderbolt Pl., Ste. E
Chantilly, VA 20151
(800)533-5503, (703)471-6400
Personal care, Cosmetics

❤ Color My Image Inc. ▧
5025B Backlick Rd.
Annadale, VA 22003
(703)354-9797
Cosmetics

❧ Color ProTec
(see Clairol, Inc.)

❤ Colora Henna ✳ ■
217 Washington Ave.
Carlstadt, NJ 07072
(201)939-0969
Personal care, Cosmetics

❤ ColorStay®
(see Revlon, Inc.)

❤ Colour Energy Corp. ✳ ■ ●
#402-55 Water St.
Vancouver, BC, V6B 1A3
Canada
(604)687-3757
Personal care

◆ Columbia Cosmetics ■
1661 Timothy Dr.
San Leandro, CA 94577
(510)562-5900
Personal care, Cosmetics

◆ Comb-Thru Texturizer
(see Pro-Line Corp.)

▼ Combat
(see Clorox Company)

▼ Comet
(see Procter & Gamble)

❤ Common Scents ● ✉
128 Main St.
Port Jefferson, NY 11777
(516)473-6370
Personal care

◆ Compassion Matters ● ✉
P.O. Box 3614
Jamestown, NY 14702-3614
(800)422-6330, (716)664-7023
*Personal care, Cosmetics,
Household, Companion animal*

❤ Concept Now Cosmetics ●
P.O. Box 3208
Santa Fe Springs, CA 90670
(562)903-1450
Cosmetics

❤ Connie Stevens/Forever Spring ●
426 S. Robertson
Los Angeles, CA 90048
(310)657-4402
Personal care, Cosmetics

❤ Consolidated Ecoprogress
Technology, Inc. ✳ ●
850 W. Hastings St., Ste. 800
Vancouver, BC, V6C 1E1
Canada
(604)801-6664
Personal care

▼ Consort Hair Spray
(see Alberto-Culver Co.)

▼ Contradiction
(see Calvin Klein Cosmetics Co.)

◆ Coolove Cool Water Wash
(see America's Finest Products Corp.)

◆ Copper Brite Inc. ✳ ■
P.O. Box 50610
Santa Barbara, CA 93150
(805)565-1566
Household

▼ Corn Huskers Lotion
(see Warner-Lambert Co.)

◆ Coronet Paper Products
(see Georgia-Pacific Corp.)

▼ Cortexx
(see Alberto-Culver Co.)

◆ Cosmair, Inc. ●
575 Fifth Ave.
New York, NY 10017
(800)631-7358, (212)818-1500
(see parent L'Oreal of Paris)
Personal care, Cosmetics

❤ Cosmetic Group, U.S.A. ●
11340 Penrose St.
Sun Valley, CA 91352
(818)767-2889
Personal care, Cosmetics

❤ Cosmetique, Inc. ● ▣
P.O. Box 94061
Palatine, IL 60094-4061
(800)621-8822, (847)913-9099
Personal care, Cosmetics

◆ Cosmyl, Inc. ■
4401 Ponce De Leon Blvd.
Coral Gables, FL 33146
(305)446-5666
Personal care, Cosmetics

◆ Cot'n Wash, Inc. ✳ ▣
502 The Times Building
Ardmore, PA 19003
(800)355-WASH, (610)896-4372
Household

▼ Cottonelle
(see Kimberly-Clark Corp.)

◆ Country Comfort ■
P.O. Box 406
Fawnskin, CA 92333-0406
(909)866-3678
Personal care

◆ Country Save Corp. ✳ ■
3410 Smith Ave.
Everett, WA 98201
(206)258-1171
Household

▼ Cover Girl Cosmetics ■
11050 York Rd.
Hunt Valley, MD 21030
(410)785-7300
(see parent Procter & Gamble)
Cosmetics

◆ Covermark Cosmetics ●
157 Veterans Dr.
Northvale, NJ 07647-2301
(201)460-7713
Cosmetics

❤ Creme de la Terre ■ ▨
30 Cook Rd.
Stamford, CT 06902
(800)260-0700, (203)324-4300
Personal care

▼ Crest
(see Procter & Gamble)

❤ Crystal Body Deodorant
(see French Transit)

❤ Crystal Candles™
(see Arizona Natural Resources, Inc.)

❤ Crystal®
(see American Safety Razor Co.)

▼ Curad
(see Colgate-Palmolive Co.)

❤ Custom Plus
(see Gillette Co.)

▼ Cutex
(see Chesebrough-Pond's USA Co.)

▼ Cyberglaze
(see Marche Image Corp.)

❤ D.K. USA, Ltd. ✳ ■
600 Old Country Rd., Room 314
Garden City, NY 11530-2010
(516)222-2250
Cosmetics

❤ Daily Essentials Body Products
(see Jafra Cosmetics Int'l)

❤ Daisy
(see Gillette Co.)

❤ Danklied Laboratories, Ltd. ✳ ■
P.O. Box 436
Cazenovia, NY 13035
(315)655-4747
Companion animal

▼ Dash
(see Procter & Gamble)

▼ Dawn
(see Procter & Gamble)

▼ d-Con
(see Reckitt & Colman)

◆ Decleor USA
18 East 48th St., 21st Fl.
New York, NY 10017
(800)722-2219, (212)838-1771
Personal care

▼ Deep Woods OFF!
(see S.C. Johnson & Son, Inc.)

▼ Degree
(see Helene Curtis Int'l)

◆ Del Laboratories, Inc. ■ ●
178 EAB Plaza
Uniondale, NY 11556
(516)844-2020
Personal care, Cosmetics

❤ Delby System ●
47 W. 34th St., Ste. 959
New York, NY 10001-3005
(212)594-5036
Personal care

❤ Delore
2220 Gaspar Ave.
City of Commerce, CA 90040
(323)728-2999
(see parent American Int'l Ind.)
Personal care, Cosmetics

❤ Dena Corp. ✳ ■
825 Nicholas Blvd.
Elk Grove Village, IL 60007
(847)593-3041
Personal care, Cosmetics

◆ Den-Mat Corp. ✳ ■
Light Years Ahead
8812 Hollywood Hills Rd.
Los Angeles, CA 90046
(800)548-3663, (323)650-2728
Personal care

◆ Dental Healthway Inc.
(formerly Oral Logic, Inc.) ✳ ■
7000 Hwy. 2 E.
Minot, ND 58701
(800)345-1143
Personal care

▼ Dentax
(see Playtex Products, Inc.)

63

♥ Deodorant Stones of
America (D.S.A.) ✳ ■
9420 East Doubletree Ranch Rd.
Scottsdale, AZ 85258
(800)666-0373, (480)451-4981
Personal care, Cosmetics

▼ Depend®
(see Kimberly-Clark Corp.)

♥ Derma E ■
9751 Independence
Chatsworth, CA 91311
(800)521-3342, (818)718-1420
Personal care

◆ Derma Guard Spray
(see Pro-Tec Pet Health)

♥ Dermafade
(see Beauty Naturally, Inc.)

♥ Derma-Glo Skin Care
(see Nutri-Cell, Inc.)

♥ Derma-Life Corp. ✳ ■
5600 McCloud NE, Ste. Q
Albuquerque, NM 87109
(505)888-1789
Personal care, Cosmetics

▼ Dermassage
(see Colgate-Palmolive Co.)

◆ Dermatone Lab Inc. ✳ ●
80 King Spring Rd.
Windsor Locks, CT 06096
(800)225-7546
Personal care

♥ Desert Pride
(see Botanical Products, Inc.)

◆ Desoto LLC ✳ ■
900 East Washington St.
Joliet, IL 60433
(815)727-4931
Household

♥ Destiny
(see Marilyn Miglin L.P.)

▼ Dettol
(see Reckitt & Colman)

◆ Devi, Inc. ✳ ■ ● ▨
P.O. Box 377
Lancaster, MA 01523
(800)BEST-221, (508)368-0066
Personal care, Cosmetics

♥ Dial Corporation, Inc. ■
15501 N. Dial Blvd.
Scottsdale, AZ 85260
(800)528-0849, (602)754-DIAL
Personal care, Household

▼ Diamond Hard Nail Enamel
(see Procter & Gamble)

▼ Diaparene
(see Playtex Products, Inc.)

❤ Dippity-Do
(see Gillette Co.)

❤ Discount Deodorant Stones ✳ ■
3503 Vara Dr.
Austin, TX 78754-4928
(800)926-5233, (512)926-9662
Personal care, Cosmetics

◆ Dish Drops® Concentrated
Dishwashing Liquid
(see Amway Corp.)

❤ Dishmate™ Dishwashing Liquid
(see Earth Friendly Products)

▼ Disney Toothbrushes
(see Chesebrough-Pond's USA Co.)

❤ DML Lotion
(see Person & Covey)

❤ Dog Poo
(see Sunfeather Natural Soap Co.)

◆ DoneGon
(see Physically Handicapped, Inc.)

❤ Donna Karan Cosmetics
(see Estee Lauder Companies)

▼ Dorothy Gray
(see Playtex Products, Inc.)

▼ Dove
(see Lever Brothers)

▼ Downy
(see Procter & Gamble)

◆ Dr. A. C. Daniels ✳ ■
109 Worcester Rd.
Webster, MA 01570-2102
(800)547-3760, (508)943-5563
Companion animal

❤ Dr. Bronner's Magic Soaps ✳ ■
P.O. Box 28
Escondido, CA 92033
(760)745-7069, (760)743-2211
Personal care, Household

❤ Dr. Bronner's Products
(see Dr. Bronner's Magic Soaps)

◆ Dr. Daniels'
(see Dr. A. C. Daniels)

❤ Dr. Goodpet ▪ ● ✉
P.O. Box 4489
Inglewood, CA 90309
(800)222-9932
Companion animal

◆ Dr. Grandel (Dr. Grandel Gmbh) ▪
32496 U.S. Hwy. 281, N.
Bulverde, TX 78613
(800)543-5230
Personal care

❤ Dr. Hauschka Cosmetics ● ✉
59C North St.
Hatfield, MA 01038
(413)247-9907
Personal care, Cosmetics

❤ Dr. Moynahan Skincare Center ●
18 Haynes St.
Hartford, CT 06103
(860)525-6200
Personal care, Cosmetics

◆ Dr. Singha's Products
(see Natural Therapeutics Centre)

❤ Dr. Willard's Catalyst Altered Water™
(see St. Clair Industries, Inc.)

◆ Drakkar Noir
(see L'Oreal of Paris)

▼ Drano
(see S.C. Johnson & Son, Inc.)

❤ Dreamous Corp. ✳ ▪ ✉
12016 Wilshire Blvd.
Los Angeles, CA 90025
(310)442-8544
Personal care, Cosmetics

▼ Dreft
(see Procter & Gamble)

❤ Dry Idea
(see Gillette Co.)

▼ Dryel Fabric Care
(see Procter & Gamble)

❤ Duck Butter™
(see Simmons Natural Bodycare)

❤ Duracell
(see Gillette Co.)

❤ Dutch® Detergent
(see Dial Corporation)

◆ Dymo
(see Essette Corp.)

❤ Dynagrip
(see Gillette Co.)

▼ Dynamo
(see Colgate-Palmolive Co.)

◆ Dyna-Vites
(see Trophy Animal Health Care)

♥ E.E. Dickinson
(see T.N. Dickinson)

▼ E.P.T. Early Pregnancy Test
(see Warner-Lambert Co.)

♥ Earth Care
(see Real Goods Trading Corp.)

♥ Earth Doctor Distributor ✳ ● ▣
828 Kings Rd.
Schenectady, NY 12303
(518)370-1904
Personal care, Household

♥ Earth Enzymes™ Drain Opener
(see Earth Friendly Products)

♥ Earth Friendly Products ✳ ▣
44 Green Bay Rd.
Winnetka, IL 60093
(800)335-ECOS, (847)446-4441
Household

◆ Earth Pack
(see MW Laboratories)

♥ Earth Science, Inc. ✳ ▣
475 N. Sheridan
Corona, CA 91720
(800)222-6720, (909)371-7505
Personal care, Cosmetics, Household

♥ Earthly Matters ✳ ▣
2950 St. Augustine Rd.
Jacksonville, FL 32207
(800)398-7503, (904)398-1458
Household

♥ Earthsafe™ Products
(see NACCO)

◆ Earthwise
(see Essette Corp.)

♥ East End Imports, Co. ▣ ▣
47 North Shore Rd., P.O. Box 107
Montauk, NY 11954
(516)668-4158
Personal care

▼ Easy-Off
(see Reckitt & Colman)

♥ Eau d'Aromes
(see Jafra Cosmetics Int'l)

♥ Eau de Parfum Falcon Spray
(see La Prairie, Inc.)

◆ Eau Pour Homme
(see L'Oreal of Paris)

💜 EB5 Corp. ● ✉
2232 E. Burnside St.
Portland, OR 97214
(503)230-8008
Cosmetics

◆ Ecco Bella ■
1133 Route 23
Wayne, NJ 07470
(201)696-7766
Personal care, Cosmetics

💜 Ecobath Soaps
(see Clearly Natural Products)

💜 Eco-Dent Int'l, Inc. ■ ● ✉
3130 Spring St.
Redwood City, CA 94063
(415)364-6343
Personal care

💜 Ecos® Laundry Detergent
(see Earth Friendly Products)

◆ Eco-Safe
(see Natural Animal, Inc.)

◆ EcoZone
(see Natural Animal, Inc.)

▼ Edge Shaving Products
(see S.C. Johnson & Son, Inc.)

▼ Efferdent
(see Warner-Lambert Co.)

◆ Elasta Products
(see Kenra, Inc.)

💜 Elephant Lube
(see Mad Gab's)

◆ ELIMINATE®
(see HERC Consumer Products)

◆ Elite Cream
(see MW Laboratories)

▼ Elizabeth Arden Co. ■
1345 Ave. of the Americas
New York, NY 10105
(212)261-1000
(see parent Unilever United
States Inc.)
Personal care, Cosmetics

▼ Elizabeth Taylor White Diamonds
(see Elizabeth Arden Co.)

❤ Elizabeth Van Buren
Aromatherapy ✳ ■
303 Potrero St., Ste. 33
Santa Cruz, CA 95060-2756
(408)425-8218
Personal care

◆ Ella Bache Beauty Products, Inc. ■ ●
8 West 36th St.
New York, NY 10018
(800)922-2430, (212)279-0842
Personal care

❤ Ellegance
(see NaturElle Cosmetics)

◆ Elysee Scientific Cosmetics ■
6804 Seybold Rd.
Madison, WI 53719
(608)271-3664
Personal care, Cosmetics

❤ Emerald Forest
(see Natural Nectar Corp.)

◆ Emporio Armani
(see L'Oreal of Paris)

◆ Energee™ Plus Shampoo
(see Espree Animal Products, Inc.)

❤ Energizer Hair Care Line
(see Hobe Laboratories, Inc.)

❤ Enviro Pet
(see Baxter Environmental Products)

❤ Eqyss Int'l ✳ ■
P.O. Box 130008
Carlsbad, CA 92013
(800)526-7469
Personal care, Companion animal

▼ Era
(see Procter & Gamble)

▼ Escape
(see Calvin Klein Cosmetics Co.)

❤ Escentual
(see Starwest Botanicals, Inc.)

❤ Espial USA Ltd. ✳ ■ ●
7045 S. Fulton St., Ste. 200
Englewood, CO 80112
(303)799-0707
Personal care, Cosmetics, Household

◆ Espree Animal Products, Inc. ■ ●
P.O. Box 167707
Irving, TX 75016
(800)328-1317
Companion animal

❤ Essence
(see Baudelaire, Inc.)

❤ Essential Purifying Gel
(see La Prairie, Inc.)

◆ Essette Corp. ✳ ■
71 Clinton Rd.
Garden City, NY 11530
Household

❤ Estee Lauder Companies, Inc. ■
767 Fifth Ave.
New York, NY 10153
(212)572-4200
Personal care, Cosmetics

▼ Eternity
(see Calvin Klein Cosmetics Co.)

❤ European Mystique Products
(see Dena Corp.)

❤ European Soaps, Ltd. ●
920 N. 137th St.
Seattle, WA 98133-7505
(206)361-9143
Personal care

❤ Eva Jon Cosmetics ✉
1016 East California St.
Gainesville, TX 76240
(817)668-7707
*Personal care, Cosmetics,
Companion animal*

◆ Ever Young, Inc. ●
55 W. Sunset Way
Issaquah, WA 98027
(425)391-1584, (425)557-4605
Personal care, Cosmetics

❤ Everybody Ltd. ● ✉
5150 Valmont Rd.
Boulder, CO 80301-2322
(800)748-5675
Personal care

▼ EverClean
(see Clorox Company)

▼ EverFresh
(see Clorox Company)

❤ Exotic Nature Body
Care Products ■ ✉
2535 Village Lane, Ste. E
Cambria, CA 93428-3428
(805)927-2517
Personal care

❤ Extra-Brite Tooth Whitener
(see Eco-Dent Int'l, Inc.)

◆ E-Z Feet Foot Balm
(see Aloette Cosmetics, Inc.)

▼ Fab
(see Colgate-Palmolive Co.)

▼ Faberge
(see Unilever United States Inc.)

◆ Face Changes
(see MW Laboratories)

💙 Face Saver
(see Gillette Co.)

💙 Face to Face ●
18399 Ventura Blvd., #10
Tarzana, CA 91356-4233
(818)881-8383
Personal care, Cosmetics

💙 Faith In Nature
(see Faith Products Ltd.)

💙 Faith Products Ltd. ■ ✉
Unit 5 Kay St.
Bury, Lancashire, BL9 6BU
England
(011)44-161-764-2555
Personal care, Household

▼ Fantastik
(see S.C. Johnson & Son, Inc.)

▼ Favor Furniture Polish
(see S.C. Johnson & Son, Inc.)

▼ FDS
(see Alberto-Culver Co.)

▼ Febreze Fabric Spray
(see Procter & Gamble)

💙 Fels Naptha® Soap
(see Dial Corporation)

💙 Female Health Company ■
875 N. Michigan Ave., Ste. 3660
Chicago, Illinois 60611
(800)884-1601
Personal care

💙 FES Products
(see Flower Essence Services)

🐛 Final Net
(see Clairol, Inc.)

▼ Final Touch
(see Lever Brothers)

▼ Fine Wood Paste Wax
(see S.C. Johnson & Son, Inc.)

▼ Finesse
(see Helene Curtis Int'l)

💙 Fire & Ice Fragrance
(see Revlon, Inc.)

▼ First Brands Corporation ■
83 Wooster Heights Rd.
Danbury, CT 06813
(203)731-2300
(see parent Clorox Company)
Household

◆ Flame Glow Cosmetics
(see Del Laboratories, Inc.)

❤ Fleabusters/Rx for Fleas ✳ ■ ● ▨
6555 NW 9th Ave., Ste. 412
Fort Lauderdale, FL 33309
(800)666-3532, (305)351-9244
Companion animal

❤ Flee Flea Oil
(see Sunfeather Natural Soap Co.)

❤ Flex
(see Revlon, Inc.)

❤ FloraSpa
(see CD&P Health Products, Inc.)

❤ Flower Essence Services ■ ▨
P.O. Box 1769
Nevada City, CA 95959
(800)548-0075, (916)265-0258
Personal care, Companion animal

❤ Flowery Beauty Products ✳ ■
P.O. Box 4008
Greenwich, CT 06830
(203)661-0995
Personal care, Cosmetics

◆ Fluff Fabric Softener
(see James Austin Co.)

❤ FM Fragrance
(see Jafra Cosmetics Int'l)

❤ Foamy Shaving Cream
(see Gillette Co.)

❤ For Pet's Sake Enterprises ✳ ● ▨
3780 Eastway Rd.
Cleveland, Ohio 44118
(800)285-0298
Personal care, Cosmetics

❤ Forest Pure
(see Levlad, Inc.)

◆ Forever New Int'l, Inc. ✳ ■
4701 N. Fourth Ave.
Sioux Falls, SD 57104-0403
(800)456-0107, (605)331-2910
Household

▼ Formula 409
(see Clorox Company)

♥ Framesi USA/Roffler ✳ ■ ●
400 Chess St.
Coraopolis, PA 15108
(412)269-2950
(see parent Styling Technology Corp.)
Personal care

♥ Frank T. Ross & Sons, Ltd. ✳ ■
6550 Lawrence Ave.
East Scarborough, Ontario
M1C 4A7, Canada
(416)282-1107
Personal care, Household

◆ Fred Hayman Beverly
Hills Fragrances
(see Parlux Fragrances, Inc.)

◆ Free Spirit Enterprises ✳ ■
P.O. Box 2638
Guerneville, CA 95446
(707)869-1942
Personal care

♥ Freeman Cosmetic Corp. ■
15501 N. Dial Blvd.
Scottsdale, AZ 85260
(480)754-3425
(see parent Dial Corporation)
Personal care, Cosmetics

♥ French Transit ✳ ■
398 Beach Rd.
Burlingame, CA 94010
(800)829-ROCK, (415)548-9600
Personal care

♥ Fresh and Natural
(see Natural Bodycare)

▼ Fresh 'n Brite
(see Warner-Lambert Co.)

▼ Fresh Start
(see Colgate-Palmolive Co.)

▼ Fresh Step Cat Litter
(see Clorox Company)

➤ Frizz Control
(see Clairol, Inc.)

◆ Fur Foam No-Rinse Pet Cleaner
(see Beaumont Products, Inc.)

▼ Future Floor Polish
(see S.C. Johnson & Son, Inc.)

♥ Gabriel Cosmetics, Inc. ✳ ■
205 108th Ave., SE
Bellevue, WA 98105
(206)688-8663
Personal care, Cosmetics

♥ Gaiam Inc. ⊠
360 Interlocken Blvd., Ste. 300
Broomfield, CO 80021
(800)869-3446
Personal care, Cosmetics, Household

▼ Gain
(see Procter & Gamble)

◆ Gannon's, Inc. ✳ ■ ⊠
1020 Seventh St.
Portsmouth, OH 45662-4105
(614)353-1667
Household, Companion animal

♥ Gap, Inc. ■
One Harrison St.
San Francisco, CA 94105
(800)333-7899, (415)952-4400
Personal care, Cosmetics

♥ Garden Botanika ■ ● ⊠
8624 154th Ave., N.E.
Redmond, WA 98052
(800)968-7842, (206)881-9603
Personal care, Cosmetics

♥ Gena Laboratories, Inc. ■
7400 E. Tierra Buena Ln.
Scottsdale, AZ 85260-1613
(480)609-6000
(see parent Styling Technology Corp.)
Personal care, Cosmetics

♥ General Therapeutics, Inc.
(see Para Laboratories, Inc.)

♥ GentleFloss Premium Dental Floss
(see Eco-Dent Int'l, Inc.)

◆ Gently Yours
(see Granny's Old Fashioned
Products)

◆ Georgette Klinger Inc. ■ ● ⊠
501 Madison Ave.
New York, NY 10022
(212)838-7080
Personal care, Cosmetics

◆ Georgia-Pacific Corp. ✳ ■
233 Peachtree St., NE, Ste. 1800
Atlanta, GA 30348-5141
(404)652-4000
Household

♥ Gerda Spillman Swiss Skin Care
(see Mar-Riche Enterprises)

♥ Germaine Monteil Cosmetics
(see Revlon, Inc.)

♥ Gillette Co. ■
Prudential Tower Building
Boston, MA 02199
(800)872-7202, (617)421-7000
Personal care, Cosmetics

▼ Giorgio Beverly Hills ■
2400 Broadway, Ste. 400
Santa Monica, CA 90404
(310)453-0711
(see parent Procter & Gamble)
Cosmetics

♥ Giovanni Hair Care Products ■
P.O. Box 39378
Los Angeles, CA 90039
(310)952-9960
Personal care, Cosmetics

▼ Glad
(see Clorox Company)

◆ Glad Rags
(see Keepers! Inc.)

▼ Glade Products
(see S.C. Johnson & Son, Inc.)

▼ Gladware
(see Clorox Company)

◆ Glass Glo
(see Pine Glo Products, Inc.)

▼ Glass Plus
(see Reckitt & Colman)

▼ Gleem Toothpaste
(see Procter & Gamble)

⧫ Glints
(see Clairol, Inc.)

◆ Glister®/Spreedent® Toothpaste
(see Amway Corp.)

▼ Glo Coat Floor Polish
(see S.C. Johnson & Son, Inc.)

◆ Global Health Alternatives ■
P.O. Box 6128
Longmont, CO 80501-2077
(800)4BE-CALM
Personal care

◆ Gloria Vanderbilt Fragrancs
(see L'Oreal of Paris)

▼ Glory Rug Cleaner
(see S.C. Johnson & Son, Inc.)

▼ Glysolid Cream
(see SmithKline Beecham
Consumer Healthcare)

◆ Gold Medal Hair Products ■ ▣
One Bennington Ave.
Freeport, NY 11520
(516)378-6900; (800)535-8101
Personal care

◆ Golden Pride Int'l ●
1501 Northpoint Pkwy., Ste. 100
West Palm Beach, FL 33407
(407)640-5700
Personal care, Cosmetics, Household

♥ Good Clean Fun
(see Smith & Vandiver)

♥ Good News
(see Gillette Co.)

◆ Goodier, Inc. ■
P.O. Box 560986
Dallas, TX 75356
(214)630-1803
Personal care

◆ Granny's Old Fashioned
Products ✳ ■
844 N. Vernon Ave. #16
Azusa, CA 91702-2254
(626)969-5066
Personal care, Household

♥ Great Mother's Goods ✳ ■ ● ⊠
501 West Fayette St., Ste. 215
Syracuse, NY 13204-2925
(315)476-1385
Personal care

♥ Green Ban ✳ ■ ●
P.O. Box 146
Norway, IA 52318
(319)446-7495
Personal care, Companion animal

◆ Groomer's Vita-Moist Hand Cream
(see Espree Animal Products, Inc.)

◆ Guy Laroche Fragrances
(see L'Oreal of Paris)

♥ H20 Plus, Inc. ●
845 W. Madison
Chicago, IL 60607
(800)242-Bath, (312)850-9283
Personal care, Cosmetics

♥ Hair Doc Co. ●
16870 Stagg St.
Van Nuys, CA 91406
(800)742-4736, (818)989-4247
Personal care, Cosmetics

♥ Hair Fitness Nutrient Hair
Care Products
(see Health and Body Fitness, Inc.)

♥ Hair Lover's
(see Hobe Laboratories, Inc.)

◆ Hair Off
(see CCA Industries, Inc.)

❤ Halsa Swedish Botanical
Hair Care Products
(see Schwarzkopf & Dep Inc.)

❤ Halston Enterprises, Inc. ◼
625 Madison Ave.
New York, NY 10022
(212)527-6770
(see parent Revlon, Inc.)
Cosmetics

❤ Halston Fragrances
(see Halston Enterprises, Inc.)

▼ Handi Wipes
(see Softsoap Enterprises)

❤ Hansen's Pet Systems
(see Kyjen Co.)

◆ Harvey Natural Citrus Cleaner
(see Specialty Products, Inc.)

❤ Hawaiian Face Products
(see Free Spirit Enterprises)

❤ Hawaiian Resources Co., Ltd. ✳ ●
94527 Puahi St.
Waipahu, HI 96797
(808)621-6270
Personal care, Cosmetics

◆ Hawaiian Tropic Products
(see Tanning Research Labs, Inc.)

▼ Head & Shoulders
(see Procter & Gamble)

❤ Health and Body Fitness, Inc. ◼
12021 Wilshire Blvd., Ste. 621
West Los Angeles, CA 90025
(562)434-6417
Personal care, Cosmetics

◆ Health From The Sun ◼
P.O. Box 840
Sunapee, NH 03782
(603)763-4745
Personal care, Cosmetics

◆ Heavenly Sheen
(see Aloette Cosmetics, Inc.)

❤ Helen Lee Skin Care &
Cosmetics ✳ ◼ ✉
205 East 60th St.
New York, NY 10022
(800)288-1077, (212)888-1233
Personal care, Cosmetics

◆ Helena Rubenstein
(see L'Oreal of Paris)

▼ Helene Curtis Int'l ■
325 N. Wells St.
Chicago, IL 60610-4713
(800)621-2013, (312)661-0222
(see parent Unilever
United States Inc.)
Personal care

◆ Henna Gold Shampoo
(see ShiKai Products)

❤ Henri Bendel, Inc. ✻ ■
712 5th Ave.
New York, NY 10019
(212)247-1100
(see parent Limited, Inc.)
Cosmetics

❤ Herb Garden ✻ ■ ● ✉
P.O. Box 773-N
Pilot Mountain, NC 27041
abeall@advi.net
Personal care, Household

◆ Herbal Armor Insect Repellent
(see All Terrain Co.)

❤ Herbal Delight
(see Dr. Hauschka
Cosmetics USA Inc.)

➤ Herbal Essences
(see Clairol, Inc.)

❤ Herbal Melange
(see Norimoor Co. Inc.)

❤ Herbal Products & Development ■
P.O. Box 1084
Aptos, CA 95001
(408)688-8706
Personal care, Household

❤ Herbal Vapors™
(see Simmons Natural Bodycare)

❤ Herbal-Glo
(see Beauty Naturally, Inc.)

❤ HerbaLife ✻
1800 Century Park, E.
Century City, CA 90067
(310)410-9600
Personal care, Cosmetics

❤ HerbalVedic Products
(see Auroma Int'l)

◆ HERC Products ✻ ■
2215 W. Melinda Ln., #A
Phoenix, AZ 85027-2629
(800)446-7448
Household

💜 Heritage Store, Inc. ■ ✉
314 Laskin Rd.
Virginia Beach, VA 23451
(800)TO-CAYCE, (757)428-0100
Personal care, Cosmetics, Household

💜 Hewitt Soap Co., Inc. ■
333 Linden Ave.
Dayton, OH 45401
(800)543-2245, (937)253-1151
(see parent American Safety
Razor Co.)
Personal care

💜 Hibiscus Collection®
(see Hewitt Soap Co., Inc.)

▼ Hi-Dri Paper Towels
(see Kimberly-Clark Corp.)

◆ High Country Cosmetics, Inc. ■
P.O. Box 280
Carbondale, CO 81623-0280
(970)704-9402
Cosmetics

◆ Hi-Lex Corp. ✳ ■ ●
990 Appolo Rd.
Eagan, MN 55121
(612)454-1160
Household

▼ Hill's Pet Nutrition, Inc. ■
400 W. 8th St.
Topeka, KS 66603
(785)354-8523
(see parent Colgate-Palmolive Co.)
Companion animal

💜 Hobe Laboratories, Inc. ✳ ■
4032 E. Broadway
Phoenix, AZ 85040
(800)528-4482
Personal care

💜 Home Service Products Co. ✳ ● ✉
P.O. Box 129
Lambertville, NJ 08530-0129
(609)397-8674
Household

💜 Homebody
(see Perfumoils, Inc.)

◆ Homesteader's Soap Co. ■
383 Kenyon Rd.
Greenwich, NY 12834-5314
Personal care

💜 Honey Silk Skin Care
(see Beehive Botanicals Inc.)

♥ Honeybee Gardens ■ ✉
P.O. Box 13
Morgantown, PA 19543-0013
(888)478-9090, (610)286-9712
Personal care

◆ Horseman's Dream ■
P.O. Box 26797
Fort Worth, TX 76126
(817)560-8818
Companion animal

♥ Hubner
(see Baudelaire, Inc.)

▼ Huggies®
(see Kimberly-Clark Corp.)

▼ Hugo Boss Fragrance
(see Procter & Gamble)

♥ Huish Detergents, Inc. ■
3540 West 1987 South
Salt Lake City, UT 84125
(800)776-6702, (801)975-3100
Household

♥ Hummers, Inc. ✳ ■ ●
HCR 32, Box 122
Uvalde, TX 78801
(830)232-6167
Personal care, Household,
Companion animal

♥ Hund-N-Flocken Dog Food Flakes
(see Solid Gold Health
Products for Pets, Inc.)

❧ Hydrience
(see Clairol, Inc.)

◆ Hydro Active
(see Dr. Grandel)

◆ Hydron Technologies, Inc. ■
1001 Yamato Rd., Ste. 403
Boca Raton, FL 33431
(800)449-3766
Personal care, Cosmetics

♥ Hyperclean
(see Zenith Is 4 The Planet)

▼ Iams
(see Procter & Gamble)

❧ Icon
(see Matrix Essentials, Inc.)

◆ Iguana
(see Amon-Re Laboratories)

◆ ILONA, INC. ■
3201 East Second Ave.
Denver, CO 80206
(888)38-ILONA
Personal care, Cosmetics

♥ Imageperfect
(see Jackie Brown Cosmetics)

♥ Imari Fragrance
(see Avon Products, Inc.)

♥ Imperial Bay Rum Fragrance
(see Deodorant Stones of
America (D.S.A.)

▼ Impressions
(see Melaleuca)

▼ Impulse Fragrance
(see Chesebrough-Pond's USA Co.)

▼ Incognito
(see Cover Girl Cosmetics)

♥ Indigo Wild Aromatics ■ ✉
6503 Summit
Kansas City, MO 64113
(800)361-5686
Personal care, Companion animal

❧ Infusium 23
(see Clairol, Inc.)

♥ Innovative Body Science ✳ ■
2724 Loker Ave. West
Carlsbad, CA 92008
(888)700-7727
Personal care

♥ Institute of Trichology ■
13918 Equitable Rd.
Cerritos, CA 90703
(800)458-8874, (562)926-7373
Personal care

♥ Internatural ✉
33719 116th St.
Twin Lakes, WI 53181
(800)643-4221
Personal care, Cosmetics, Household

♥ Inverness Corp. ✳ ■
17-10 Willow St.
Fair Lawn, NJ 07410
(800)524-1303, (201)794-3400
Personal care

▼ Irish Spring
(see Colgate-Palmolive Co.)

▼ Ironclad Finish
(see Marche Image Corp.)

◆ Irving Tissue, Inc. ✳ ■
International Plaza II, Ste. 322
Philadelphia, PA 19113
(800)952-6633, (610)362-0800
Personal care

♥ Island Dog ✳ ■
3 Milltown Ct.
Union, NJ 0783
(800)456-ISLAND
Personal care, Cosmetics

♥ Island Pup
(see Island Dog)

▼ Ivory
(see Procter & Gamble)

♥ Izy's Aromatherapy Skin Care
& Holistic Cosmetics ✳ ■ ● ✉
13399 Terry
Detroit, MI 48227
(313)836-2675
Personal care, Cosmetics

♥ J & J Jojoba/California
Gold Products ✳ ■ ● ✉
7826 Timm Rd.
Vacaville, CA 95688
(707)447-1207
Personal care, Cosmetics

♥ J. Stephen Scherer, Inc. ■
P.O. Box 214497
Auburn Hills, MI 48321
(810)852-8500
Cosmetics

◆ J.R. Liggett Ltd. ✳ ■
RR 2, Box 911, Route 12-A
Cornish, NH 03745
(603)675-2055
Personal care

♥ Jackie Brown Cosmetics ■
5121 Gordon Smith Dr.
Rowlett, TX 75088
(800)756-6138
Personal care, Cosmetics

♥ Jacki's Magic Lotion ■
258 A St., #7-A
Ashland, OR 97520
(541)488-1388
Cosmetics

▼ Jaclyn Smith's California
(see Procter & Gamble)

♥ Jafra Cosmetics Int'l ■
P.O. Box 5026
West Lake Valley, CA 91359
(805)449-3000
Personal care, Cosmetics

◆ James Austin Co. ■
P.O. Box 827
Mars, PA 16046-0827
(800)245-1942, (412)625-1535
Household

- ❤ Jamieson Laboratories ■ ●
  2 St. Clair Ave., West, 16th Fl.
  Toronto, Ontario, M4V 1L5
  Canada
  (416)960-0052
  Personal care, Cosmetics

- ❤ Janene Int'l, Inc. ✳ ▣
  8604 2nd Ave., #147
  Silver Spring, MD 20910
  (800)480-3153
  Personal care

- ❤ Janta Int'l Co. (J. I. C.) ✳ ●
  P.O. Box 623
  Belmont, CA 94002-0623
  (650)591-9465
  Personal care, Cosmetics

- ❤ Jasmine Natural
  (see Kyjen Co.)

- ❤ Jason Natural Products ■
  8468 Warner Dr.
  Culver City, CA 90232
  (800)527-6605, (310)838-7543
  Personal care

- ▼ Javex Liquid Bleach
  (see Colgate-Palmolive Co.)

- ❧ Jazzing
  (see Clairol, Inc.)

- ❤ JC Garet, Inc. ✳ ■ ●
  2471 Coral St.
  Vista, CA 92083
  (800)548-9770, (760)598-0505
  Household

- ❤ Jean Michelle
  (see Cosmetique, Inc.)

- ❤ Jean Nate
  (see Revlon, Inc.)

- ❤ Jeanne Gatineau Fragrance
  (see Revlon, Inc.)

- ❤ Jelene (Cosmetic Research Corp.) ■
  1332 Anderson Rd., Ste. 115
  Clawson, MI 48017-1044
  (248)435-2446
  Personal care, Cosmetics

- ❤ Jelmar, Inc. ✳ ■ ●
  6600 N. Lincoln Ave.
  Lincolnwood, IL 60645
  (847)675-8400
  Household

- ❤ Jeremy Rose Skin Care
  (see New Chapter, Inc.)

- ❤ JF9 Fragrance
  (see Jafra Cosmetics Int'l)

▼ Jhirmack Hair Care Products
(see Playtex Products, Inc.)

❤ Jobmaster
(see Huish Detergents, Inc.)

❤ John Amico Expressive
Hair Care Products ■
4731 136th St.
Crestwood, IL 60445-1968
(708)824-4000
Personal care

❤ John Frieda Professional
Hair Care, Inc. ■
57 Danbury Rd.
Wilton, CT 06897
(800)521-3189, (203)762-1233
Personal care

◆ John O. Butler Co. ✳ ■
4635 W. Foster Ave.
Chicago, IL 60630
(773)777-4000
Personal care

❤ John Paul Mitchell Systems ✳ ■
26455 Golden Valley Rd.
Saugus, CA 91350
(805)298-0400
Personal care

▼ Johnson & Johnson ■
One Johnson & Johnson Plaza
New Brunswick, NJ 08933
(908)524-3348
Personal care

▼ Johnson's Baby Oil
(see Johnson & Johnson)

▼ Johnson's Baby Powder
(see Johnson & Johnson)

❤ JOICO Labs, Inc. ✳ ■
345 Baldwin Park Blvd.
City of Industry, CA 91746
(800)445-6426, (626)968-6111
Personal care

❤ joie de vivre Fragrance
(see Jafra Cosmetics Int'l)

◆ Jolen Creme Bleach Corp. ✳ ■
P.O. Box 458
Fairfield, CT 06430
(203)259-8779
Personal care, Companion animal

▼ Jonny Cat
(see Clorox Company)

❤ Jontue
(see Revlon, Inc.)

▼ Joy
(see Procter & Gamble)

💜 Joyspray 888 Skin Refresher
(see Janta Int'l Co. (J.I.C.))

◆ JPR3
(see CCA Industries, Inc.)

▼ Jubilee Spray
(see S.C. Johnson & Son, Inc.)

◆ Just for Me!
(see Pro-Line Corp.)

◆ Just 'N Time Stain Remover
(see SerVaas Laboratories Inc.)

🌶 Kaleidocolors
(see Clairol, Inc.)

◆ Karpet Kleen
(see Granny's Old
Fashioned Products)

💜 Katz-N-Flocken
(see Solid Gold Health
Products for Pets, Inc.)

◆ Keepers! Inc. ✳ ■ ▨
P.O. Box 12648
Portland, OR 97212
(800)799-4523
Personal care

◆ Kenra, Inc. ■
6501 Julian Ave.
Indianapolis, IN 46219
(317)356-6491
Personal care

💜 Kensington Selection®
(see Hewitt Soap Co., Inc.)

🌶 Keri
(see Bristol-Myers Squibb Co.)

💜 Kettle Care ■ ▨
6590 Farm to Market Rd.
Whitefish, MT 59937-8301
(406)892-3294
Personal care, Household

◆ Key West Fragrance &
Cosmetic Factory, Inc. ■ ● ▨
P.O. Box 1079
Key West, FL 30401-1079
(800)445-ALOE, (305)294-5592
*Personal care, Cosmetics,
Companion animal*

◆ Keystone Laboratories, Inc. ■
P.O. Box 2026
Memphis, TN 38101
(901)774-8860
Personal care

💜 Khepra Skin Care, Inc. ■
3939 IDS Center, 80 S. Eighth St.
Minneapolis, MN 55402
(612)823-5656
Personal care

💜 Kiehl's ■ ● ▣
109 Third Ave.
New York, NY 10003
(212)677-3171
Personal care, Cosmetics

💜 Kim Manley Herbals ■
7200 Panoramic Hwy.
Stinston Beach, CA 94970
(415)868-0825
Personal care

▼ Kimberly-Clark Corp. ■
P.O. Box 619100
Dallas, TX 75261-9100
(800)544-1847, (972)281-1200
Personal care

▼ Kingsford Products Company ■
1221 Broadway St.
Oakland, CA 94612
(510)271-7000
(see parent Clorox Company)
Household

▼ Kirkman Soap Products
(see Colgate-Palmolive Co.)

💜 Kiss My Face Corp. ■
P.O. Box 224
Gardiner, NY 12525-0224
(800)262-KISS, (914)255-0884
Personal care, Cosmetics

▼ Klean 'n Shine
(see S.C. Johnson & Son, Inc.)

◆ Kleen Brite Labs, Inc. ■
200 State St.
Brockport, NY 14420-2028
(800)800-6370
Household

▼ Kleen Guard
(see Alberto-Culver Co.)

▼ Kleenex®
(see Kimberly-Clark Corp.)

▼ Kleenite Denture Cleaner
(see Procter & Gamble)

◆ KMS Research, Inc. ■
P.O. Box 496040
Redding, CA 96049-6040
(800)DIALKMS, (530)244-6000
Personal care

◆ Kneipp Corp. of America ✳ ●
105 Stonehurst Ct., Ste. 2
Northvale, NJ 07647-2405
(800)937-4372, (201)750-0600
Personal care

❤ Knowing
(see Estee Lauder Companies)

❤ Kolestral
(see Wella)

▼ Kotex®
(see Kimberly-Clark Corp.)

◆ Kryolan Corp. ■ ●
132 Ninth St.
San Francisco, CA 94103
(415)863-9684
Cosmetics

❤ KSA Jojoba ✳ ■
19025 Parthenia St.
Northridge, CA 91324
(818)701-1534
Personal care, Cosmetics,
Companion animal

❤ Kyjen Co. ✳ ■
P.O. Box 793
Huntington Beach, CA 92648
(800)477-5735, (714)704-1790
Household, Companion animal

❤ L'anza Research International ■
935 W. 8th St.
Azusa, CA 90172
(800)423-0307
Personal care

◆ L.O.C.® Multi-Purpose Cleaner
(see Amway Corp.)

◆ L'Oreal of Paris ■
41 Rue Martare
92110 Clichy, Cedex, France
01-47-56-7000
Personal care, Cosmetics

▼ La Coupe
(see Playtex Products, Inc.)

❤ La Crista, Inc. ✳ ■ ●
P.O. Box 240
Davidsonville, MD 21035
(800)888-2231, (410)956-4447
Personal care, Cosmetics

◆ La Cross ■
565 Broad Hollow Rd.
Farmingdale, NY 11735
(516)293-7070
(see parent Del Laboratories, Inc.)
Personal care

♥ La Dove, Inc. ■
16100 NW 48th Ave.
Hialeah, FL 33014
(305)624-2456
Personal care

♥ La France® Brightener
(see Dial Corporation)

♥ LA Looks Hair Care
(see Schwarzkopf & Dep Inc.)

◆ La Natura ✳ ■ ● ✉
425 N. Bedford Dr.
Beverly Hills, CA 90210-4302
(800)352-6288, (310)271-5616
Personal care

♥ La Prairie, Inc. ✳ ■ ●
31 West 52nd St.
New York, NY 10019-6118
(212)459-1600
Personal care, Cosmetics

◆ La Viola Dry Skin Creme
(see High Country Cosmetics)

◆ Laboratories Garnier ■
33 rue Martre
F-92117 Clichy, France
01-47-59-8122
(see parent L'Oreal of Paris)
Personal care

◆ Lady Burd Exclusive Private
Label Cosmetics ■
44 Executive Blvd.
Farmingdale, NY 11735
(516)454-0444
Cosmetics

◆ Lady Love Skin Care ■
1501 Northpoint Parkway, Ste. 100
West Palm Beach, FL 33407
(561)640-5700
(see parent Golden Pride Int'l)
Personal care

♥ Lady Mitchum
(see Revlon, Inc.)

♥ Lady of the Lake Co. ✳ ■ ✉
P.O. Box 7140
Brookings, OR 97415
(503)469-3354
Personal care

♥ Lady Personna
(see American Safety Razor Co.)

▼ Lady Speed Stick
(see Mennen Co.)

▼ Lagerfeld
(see Elizabeth Arden Co.)

▼ Lagerfeld Jako
(see Elizabeth Arden Co.)

♥ Lakon Herbals ■
RR 1, Box 4710
Montpelier, VT 05602
(802)223-5563
Personal care

♥ Lancaster Inc. ■
767 Fifth Ave.
New York, NY 10153
(212)572-5000
(see parent Revlon, Inc.)
Cosmetics

◆ Lancome
(see L'Oreal of Paris)

♥ Lanex Hemorrhoid Creme
(see Carma Laboratories, Inc.)

◆ Lange Products, Inc. ■
21093 Forbes Ave.
Hayward, CA 94545
(510)785-2177
Personal care, Cosmetics

♥ Lan-O-Sheen, Inc. ■ ●
301 County Rd., E2 W
St. Paul, MN 55112-6859
(651)645-2270
Personal care, Household

▼ Lasting Color Lipstick
(see Procter & Gamble)

◆ Lasting Pride Cat Litter
(see Oil-Dri Corporation
of America)

♥ Lauder for Men
(see Estee Lauder Companies)

▼ Laura Biagiotti-Roma Fragrance
(see Procter & Gamble)

◆ Lauren by Ralph Lauren
(see L'Oreal of Paris)

▼ Lava
(see Procter & Gamble)

♥ Lavilin
(see Beauty Naturally, Inc.)

♥ Lavoris Oral Rinse
(see Schwarzkopf & Dep Inc.)

♥ Le Crystal Naturel
(see French Transit)

▼ le Jardin
(see Procter & Gamble)

♥ le moire
(see Jafra Cosmetics Int'l)

89

❤ Legend Fragrance
(see Jafra Cosmetics Int'l)

❤ LegMate Therapy™
(see American Safety Razor Co.)

❤ Les Femmes, Inc. ✳ ■ ●
17890 Isle Ave., Ste #100
Lakeville, MN 55044
(612)892-7990
Personal care

◆ Leslie Dee Ann Cosmetics
(see Neways Int'l)

▼ Lestoil
(see Clorox Company)

▼ Lever 2000
(see Lever Brothers)

▼ Lever Brothers Co. ■
800 Sylvan Ave.
Englewood Cliffs, NJ 07632
(800)598-1223
(see parent Unilever United States, Inc.)
Personal care, Household

❤ Levlad, Inc./Nature's Gate ✳ ■
9200 Mason Ave.
Chatsworth, CA 91311
(800)327-2012, (818)882-2951
Personal care

❤ Liberty Natural Products, Inc. ●
8120 S.E. Stark St.
Portland, OR 97215
(800)289-8427, (503)256-1227
Personal care

◆ Life Changes Plus
(see MW Laboratories)

❤ Life Tree Products
(see Sierra Dawn Products)

▼ Lifebuoy
(see Lever Brothers)

❤ Lifeline Company ✳ ■
P.O. Box 531
Fairfax, CA 94930
(415)457-9024
Household

▼ Lightdays
(see Kimberly-Clark Corp.)

❤ Liken®
(see Earth Science, Inc.)

❤ Lilt
(see Schwarzkopf & Dep Inc.)

♥ Lily of Colorado ■ ● ⊠
P.O. Box 12471
Denver, CO 80212
(800)333-5459, (303)455-4194
Personal care, Cosmetics

♥ Limited, Inc. ■
Three Limited Pkwy.
P.O. Box 16528
Columbus, OH 43216
(614)479-7000
Personal care, Cosmetics

♥ Linda Seidel Transforming
Cosmetics ✳ ●
2328 W. Joppa Rd., Ste. 100
Lutherville, MD 21093-4668
(800)752-0066, (800)590-5335
Cosmetics

◆ Lip Colour Modifier
(see Aloette Cosmetics, Inc.)

◆ Lip Difference
(see Aloette Cosmetics, Inc.)

♥ Lip Gear
(see Bonne Bell, Inc.)

♥ Lip Lix
(see Bonne Bell, Inc.)

♥ Lip Lube
(see Mad Gab's)

◆ Lip Savvy
(see Strong Skin Savvy)

♥ Lip Smackers
(see Bonne Bell, Inc.)

♥ Lip Trip
(see Mountain Ocean)

♥ Lipservice Facial Hair Removal
(see Les Femmes)

♥ Liquid Dial®
(see Dial Corporation)

♥ Liquid Paper
(see Gillette Co.)

▼ Liquid Plumr
(see Clorox Company)

♥ Lissa's Garden
(see Exotic Nature Body
Care Products)

▼ Listerine
(see Warner-Lambert Co.)

▼ Listermint
(see Warner-Lambert Co.)

❤ Little Forest Natural
Baby Products ✳ ◼
2415 3rd St., Ste. 238
San Francisco, CA 94107
(415)621-6504
Personal care

❤ Living Earth Bath Treatment
(see Norimoor, Inc.)

❤ Living Nail
(see Arizona Natural
Resources, Inc.)

◆ Liz Claiborne Cosmetics ✳ ◼
1441 Broadway
New York, NY 10018
(212)354-4900
Personal care, Cosmetics

◆ Lobob Laboratories, Inc. ✳ ◼
1440 Atteberry Lane
San Jose, CA 95131-1410
(800)835-6262, (408)432-0580
Personal care

❧ Logics
(see Matrix Essentials, Inc.)

❤ Logodent
(see Logona USA, Inc.)

❤ Logona USA, Inc. ◼
554-E Riverside Dr.
Asheville, NC 28801
(800)648-6654, (828)252-1420
Personal care, Cosmetics

❤ Lord & Berry Cosmetics
(see AM Cosmetics, Inc.)

❤ Lotions & Potions ● ▣
406 S. Rockford Dr., Ste. 6
Tempe, AZ 85281
(800)462-7595, (408)968-4662
Personal care

❤ Lotus Brands ✳ ◼
P.O. Box 325
Twin Lakes, WI 53181
(800)478-6378, (262)889-8501
Personal care, Cosmetics

❤ Lotus Light Enterprises ●
P.O. Box 1008
Silver Lake, WI 53170
(800)548-3824, (262)889-8501
*Personal care, Cosmetics,
Household, Companion animal*

❤ Lotus Pads ✳ ◼ ▣
131 NW Fourth, Ste. 156
Corvallis, OR 97330
503-758-4110
Personal care

❤ Louise Bianco Skin Care, Inc. ● ⊠
13655 Chandler Blvd.
Sherman Oaks, CA 91401
(800)782-3067, (818)786-2700
Personal care, Cosmetics

❥ Loving Care
(see Clairol, Inc.)

❤ LPI, Inc. ●
535 5th Ave., Fl. 17
New York, NY 10017-3610
(800)277-6511, (212)856-9700
Cosmetics

▼ Lubriderm
(see Warner-Lambert Co.)

❤ Luminescence Catalog ●
P.O. Box 2364
Maple Plain, MN 55592
(800)364-6637, (888)676-9646
*Personal care, Cosmetics,
Household*

❤ Lunar Farms Herbal Specialist ■
3 Highland Dr.
Gilmer, TX 75644
(903)734-5893
Personal care

▼ Luster Products, Inc. ■
1104 West 43rd St.
Chicago, IL 60609
(773)579-1800
Personal care, Cosmetics

▼ Luvs
(see Procter & Gamble)

▼ Lux
(see Unilever United States Inc.)

◆ Luxury Remoisturizer
(see Espree Animal Products, Inc.)

◆ Luxury Tar & Sulfa Shampoo
(see Espree Animal Products, Inc.)

◆ Luzier Personalized Cosmetics ■ ● ⊠
3216 Gillham Plaza
Kansas City, MO 64109
(816)531-8338
Personal care, Cosmetics

▼ Lysol
(see Reckitt & Colman)

❤ MAC Cosmetics ■
233 Carlton St., #201
Toronto, Ontario M5A 2L2
Canada
(800) 387-6707, (416)924-0598
(see parent Estee Lauder Companies)
Cosmetics

93

▼ MACH3
(see Gillette Co.)

♥ Mad Gab's ■
P.O. Box 5207
Portland, ME 04101-0907
(207)772-3117
Cosmetics

◆ Magic Mountain
(see Surco Products, Inc.)

♥ Magic of Aloe, Inc. ■ ● ✉
7300 N. Crescent Blvd.
Pennsauken, NJ 08110
(800)257-7770, (856)662-3334
Personal care, Cosmetics

▼ Magic Sizing Starch
(see Church & Dwight Co., Inc.)

◆ Magick Baby
(see Magick Botanicals)

◆ Magick Botanicals ✳ ■
3412 W. MacArthur Blvd., Ste. K
Santa Ana, CA 92704
(800)237-0674, (714)957-0674
Personal care

♥ Maharishi Ayur-Veda
Products ■ ● ✉
1068 Elkton Dr.
Colorado Springs, CO 80907
(719)260-5500
Personal care

◆ Maine Mountain Soap & Candle ■
P.O. Box 130, Main St.
Greenville, ME 04441-0130
(800)287-2141
Personal care, Companion animal

♥ Mallory Pet Supplies ✳ ■
118 Atrisco Dr., SW
Albuquerque, NM 87105
(505)836-4033
Companion animal

◆ Mandarin Vanilla Fragrance
(see CCA Industries, Inc.)

◆ Maple Hill Farm ■ ✉
1224 33rd St.
Allegan, MI 49010
(616)673-6346
Personal care

♥ Marcal Paper Mills, Inc. ✳ ■ ●
1 Market St.
Elmwood Park, NJ 07407
(201)796-4000
Household

▼ Marche Image Corp. ■
P.O. Box 1010
Bronxville, NY 10708
(800)753-9980, (914)793-2093
Personal care, Household

❤ Margarite Cosmetics/Moon
Products, Inc. ✳ ■
2138 Okeechobee Blvd.
West Palm Beach, FL 33409
(561)686-1466
Cosmetics

❤ Marilyn Miglin, L.P. ■ ● ▨
127 W. Huron
Chicago, IL 60610
(800)662-1120, (312)266-4600
Personal care, Cosmetics

◆ Mario Badescu Skin Care, Inc. ■
320 E. 52nd St.
New York, NY 10022
(800)BADESCU, (212)758-1065
Personal care, Cosmetics

❤ Mar-Riche Enterprises, Inc. ■ ●
640 Glass Lane
Modesto, CA 95356
(209)529-1757
Personal care, Cosmetics

◆ Mary Ellen
Products, Inc. ✳ ■ ● ▨
Box 39221
Minneapolis, MN 55439
(612)941-1233
Household

❤ Mary Kay Cosmetics, Inc. ■
16251 Dallas Pkwy.
Dallas, TX 75248-2696
(800)MARYKAY, (972)687-6300
Personal care, Cosmetics

▼ Massengill Feminine
Hygiene Products
(see SmithKline Beecham
Consumer Healthcare)

❤ Master's Flower Essences ✳ ■ ▨
14618 Tyler Foote Rd.
Nevada City, CA 95959-9316
(800)347-3639, (530)478-7655
Personal care, Companion animal

❤ Mastey De Paris, Inc. ✳ ■
25413 Rye Canyon Rd.
Valencia, CA 91355
(800)6MASTEY, (661)257-4814
Personal care, Cosmetics

▼ Mate
(see Melaleuca)

◆ Matrix Essentials, Inc. ■
30601 Carter St.
Solon, OH 44139
(800)282-2822, (440)248-3700
(see parent Bristol-Myers
Squibb Co.)
Personal care

▼ Max Factor Cosmetics
(see Procter & Gamble)

◆ Maybelline, Inc. ■
575 Fifth Ave.
New York, NY 10017
(212)818-1500
(see parent L'Oreal of Paris)
Cosmetics

❤ McAuley's Inc. ✳ ■
2300 Sitler St.
Memphis, TN 38114
(901)946-8800
Personal care, Household

◆ McWolf Enterprises ✳ ■
125 Noble St.
Norristown, PA 19401
(800)298-SUN1, (800)596-7233
Household

◆ MD Bath Tissue
(see Georgia-Pacific Corp.)

◆ Mean Green Super Strength
Cleaners
(see Chem Pro)

◆ Medicine Flower ✳ ■
720 NE Granger Ave., Ste. A
Corvallis, OR 97330-9660
(541)745-3055
Personal care, Cosmetics

❤ MediPatch Laboratories
Corp. ✳ ■ ● ▣
P.O. Box 795
E. Dennis, MA 02641
(508)385-4549
Companion animal

❤ Megas®
(see American Safety Razor Co.)

◆ Melacaid™ Shampoo
(see Espree Animal Products, Inc.)

▼ Melaleuca, Inc. ■
3910 S. Yellowstone
Idaho Falls, ID 83402
(888)528-2090, (208)522-0700
*Personal care, Cosmetics,
Household, Companion animal*

▼ Mennen Company ■
300 Park Ave.
New York, NY 10022
(212)310-2000
(see parent Colgate-Palmolive Co.)
Personal care

▼ Mentadent
(see Chesebrough-Pond's USA Co.)

♥ Mera Personal Care
Products ✳ ■ ● ✉
P.O. Box 218
Circle Pines, MN 55014
(800)752-7261
Personal care

♥ Mere Cie Inc. ✳ ●
1100 Soscol Ferry Rd., #3
Napa, CA 94558
(800)832-4544, (707)257-8510
Personal care

♥ Mer-Flu-An
(see Eco-Dent Int'l, Inc.)

♥ Merle Norman Cosmetics ■
9130 Bellanca Ave.
Los Angeles, CA 90045
(800)421-2060, (310)641-3000
Personal care, Cosmetics

▼ Mersene Denture Cleaner
(see Colgate-Palmolive Co.)

♥ Meta Int'l, Inc. ■
825 Nicholas Blvd.
Elk Grove Village, IL 60007
(847)593-3044
Personal care, Cosmetics

♥ Mia Rose Products, Inc. ✳ ■
177-F Riverside Ave.
Newport Beach, CA 92663
(800)292-6339, (714)662-5465
Household

♥ Michael's Naturopathic Programs ■
6203 Woodlake Center
San Antonio, TX 78244
(800)525-9643, (210)661-8311
Personal care

♥ Mint Foot Masage Cream
(see Exotic Nature Body
Care Products)

♥ Mitchum
(see Revlon, Inc.)

♥ MoistStic
(see Real Natural Products, Inc.)

◆ Moisture Guard
(see Granny's Old
Fashioned Products)

▼ Moisture Rich Lipstick
(see Procter & Gamble)

❤ Moisture Therapy
(see Avon Products, Inc.)

❧ Moisturel
(see Bristol-Myers Squibb Co.)

❤ Monoi Cosmetics
(see Jason Natural Products)

◆ Monoi Tiare Tahiti Coconut Oil
(see Hawaiian Resources Co., Ltd.)

❤ Montagne Jeunesse ■
The Old Grain Store, 4 Denne Rd.
Horsham, West Sussex
RH12 1JE, England
011-44-81-877-3227
Personal care, Cosmetics

◆ Montego Bay Sachets
(see Beaumont Products, Inc.)

◆ Mood Magic Lipstick
(see CCA Industries, Inc.)

▼ Mop & Glo
(see Reckitt & Colman)

❤ Moriah Dead Sea Bath Salts
(see Colora Henna)

❤ Morrill's New Directions ▨
21 Market Sq.
Houlton, ME 04730
(800)368-5057
*Personal care, Cosmetics,
Companion animal*

❤ Motherlove herbal company ■ ▨
P.O. Box 101, 3101 Kintzley Plaza
Laporte, CO 80535-0101
(970)493-2892
Personal care

❤ Mother's Fragrances Oils
(see Mere Cie, Inc.)

◆ Mother's Little Miracle, Inc. ✳ ■
27520 Hawthorne Blvd, Ste. 125
Rolling Meadows, CA 90274
(310)544-7125
*Personal care, Household,
Companion animal*

❤ Mother's Special Blend
(see Mountain Ocean)

▼ Motions Hair Products
(see Alberto-Culver Co.)

❤ Mountain Dog
(see Island Dog)

❤ Mountain Ocean Ltd. ■
5150 Valmont Rd.
Boulder, CO 80301
(303)444-2781
Personal care, Cosmetics

❤ Mountain Rose Herbs ■ ▣
20818 High St.
North San Juan, CA 95960
(800)879-3337
*Personal care, Cosmetics,
Companion animal*

❤ Mr. Aloe Skin Care Products
(see The Magic of Aloe, Inc.)

▼ Mr. Bubble
(see Playtex Products, Inc.)

▼ Mr. Clean
(see Procter & Gamble)

❤ Murad, Inc. ✳ ■
2121 Rosecrans Ave., 5th Fl.
El Segundo, CA 90245
(800)242-1103
Personal care, Cosmetics

▼ Murphy-Phoenix Co. ■
25800 Science Park Dr.
Beachwood, OH 44122
(800)486-7627
(see parent Colgate-Palmolive Co.)
Household

▼ Murphy's Oil Soap
(see Murphy-Phoenix Co.)

◆ MW Laboratories ■ ▣
2002 52nd St. Extension
Savannah, GA 31405
(912)236-9430
*Personal care, Cosmetics,
Companion animal*

❤ Mystic
(see Marilyn Miglin L.P.)

◆ N.Y.C. New York Color Cosmetics
(see Del Laboratories, Inc.)

❤ NAACO ✳ ■
15600 New Century Dr.
Gardena, CA 90248
(310)515-1700
Household

❤ Nadina's Cremes ■ ● ▣
3813 Middletown Branch Rd.
Vienna, MD 21869-1533
(800)722-4292, (410)901-1052
Personal care, Cosmetics

❤ Nail Gear
(see Bonne Bell, Inc.)

❤ Nala Barry Labs
(see Baxter Environmental Products)

99

❤ Native Scents, Inc. ■ ✉
Box 5639
Toas, NM 87571
(800)645-3471, (505)758-9656
Personal care

❤ Natracare ✻ ■
191 University Blvd., Ste. 294
Denver, CO 80206
(303)320-1510
Personal care

❤ NaturActives
(see Starwest Botanicals, Inc.)

◆ Natural Animal, Inc. ■
7000 US 1 N., P.O. Box 1177
St. Augustine, FL 32095
(800)274-7387, (904)824-5884
Companion animal

❤ Natural Beginnings®
(see Hewitt Soap Co., Inc.)

❤ Natural Bodycare ✻ ■
355 N. Lantana St., Ste. 574
Camarillo, CA 93010-9657
(805)445-9237
Personal care, Household

❤ Natural Dentist
(see Woodstock Natural
Products, Inc.)

➤ Natural Instincts
(see Clairol, Inc.)

❤ Natural Nectar Corp. ■
2200 Vesper Circle, Ste. F5
Corona, CA 91719-3526
(909)372-2606
Personal care

◆ Natural Research
People Inc. ✻ ■ ● ✉
S. Route, Box 12
Lavina, MT 59046
(406)575-4343
Companion animal

❤ Natural Solutions Stain
& Odor Remover
(see Kyjen Co.)

◆ Natural Therapeutics
Centre ✻ ■ ● ✉
2500 Side Cove
Austin, TX 78704
(512)444-2862
Personal care, Household

◆ Natural Way Natural
Body Care ✻ ✉
820 Massachusetts St.
Lawrence, KS 66044
(785)841-8100
Personal care, Cosmetics

◆ Naturally Beautiful ⌧
P.O. Box 6329
Santa Rosa, CA 95406
(800)440-7285, (707)542-4149
*Personal care, Cosmetics,
Companion animal*

◆ Naturally Best Herbal Pet Products
(see Natural Research People Inc.)

♥ Naturally Fresh Deodorant
Crystal
(see TCCD Int'l)

♥ Nature Clean Products
(see Frank T. Ross & Sons, Ltd.)

♥ Nature de France, Ltd.
(see Para Laboratories, Inc.)

♥ NaturElle Cosmetics Corp. ✳ ■ ● ⌧
P.O. Box 3848
Telluride, CO 81435-3848
(800)442-3936
Personal care, Cosmetics

♥ Nature's Accent®
(see Dial Corporation)

◆ Nature's Acres ■ ⌧
East 8984 Weinke Rd.
North Freedom, WI 53951
(608)522-4492
Personal care

♥ Nature's Apothacary ■
1558 Cherry St.
Louisville, CO 80027
(800)999-7422
Personal care

♥ Nature's Family Skin
Care Products
(see Schwarzkopf & Dep Inc.)

♥ Nature's Gate
(see Levlad, Inc.)

♥ Nature's Key
(see American Eco-Systems)

♥ Nature's Radiance ■ ● ⌧
23704-5 El Toro Rd., PMB #513
Lake Forest, CA 92630
(877)628-8736, (949)588-9438
Personal care

◆ Nature's ScienCeuticals
(see Neways Int'l)

♥ Nature's Sunshine
Products, Inc. ■ ●
P.O. Box 19005, 75 E. 1700 S
Provo, UT 84605-9005
(801)342-4300
Personal care

♥ Nature's WEALTH ✳ ⬚
2401 W. White Oaks Dr.
Springfield, IL 62704
(800)587-6288
Personal care

♥ NatureWorks Inc.
(see Abkit, Inc.)

◆ Naturistics® Products ■
565 Broad Hollow Rd.
Farmingdale, NY 11735
(516)293-7070
(see parent Del Laboratories, Inc.)
Personal care, Cosmetics

♥ Naturpathics®
(see Earth Science, Inc.)

▼ Navy
(see Cover Girl Cosmetics)

◆ Nectarine
(see AKA Saunders, Inc.)

◆ Neem
(see Espree Animal Products, Inc.)

▼ Neet
(see Reckitt & Colman)

♥ Neo Tech Cosmetic, Inc. ■
20600 Belshaw Ave.
Carson, CA 90746
(800)432-3787, (310)898-1630
Personal care, Household

♥ Nettie Rosenstein Fragrances
(see Classic Fragrances Ltd.)

🐾 Neutrogena Corp. ■
5760 W. 96th St.
Los Angeles, CA 90045-5544
(800)421-6857, (310)642-1150
(see parent Johnson & Johnson)
Personal care

♥ New Beginnings
(see Natural Bodycare)

♥ New Chapter, Inc. ✳ ■
P.O. Box 1947
Brattleboro, VT 05302
(800)543-7279, (802)254-0390
Personal care

▼ New Definition Perfecting Make-Up
(see Procter & Gamble)

◆ New Derm Labs, Inc. ● ⬚
P.O. Box 411057
Los Angeles, CA 90041
(626)440-9933
Personal care

▼ New Freedom
(see Kimberly-Clark Corp.)

💜 New Methods ✳ ●
P.O. Box 22605
San Francisco, CA 94122
(415)379-9065
Companion animal

◆ Neways Int'l ■
150 E. 400 N., P.O. Box 651
Salem, UT 84653-0651
(800)799-5656, (801)423-2800
*Personal care, Cosmetics,
Household*

◆ NewBrite Products
(see Neways Int'l)

💜 Nexxus Products Co. ■ ●
P.O. Box 1274
Santa Barbara, CA 93116
(800)444-6399, (805)968-6900
Personal care

❧ Nice 'n Easy
(see Clairol, Inc.)

💜 Nirvana Inc. ✳ ■ ●
P.O. Box 26275
Minneapolis, MN 55426
(800)432-2919, (619)932-2919
(see parent Lotus Brands)
Personal care

💜 Nitro, Stages, Jolt ✳ ■
33 SE Eleventh St.
Grand Rapids, MN 55744
(800)556-4876, (218)326-0281
Personal care

▼ No More Tears
(see Johnson & Johnson)

💜 No Sweat
(see Revlon, Inc.)

◆ NO-AD Products
(see Solor Cosmetic Labs, Inc.)

◆ Norelco Consumer Products Co. ■
High Ridge Park, P.O. Box 10166
Stamford, CT 06912-0015
(203)973-0200
Personal care

💜 Norell Perfumes, Inc. ■
767 Fifth Ave.
New York, NY 10153
(212)572-5000
(see parent Revlon, Inc.)
Cosmetics

💜 Norimoor Co., Inc. ✳ ■ ●
3801 23rd Ave.
Long Island City, NY 11105
(212)695-6667
*Personal care, Cosmetics,
Companion animal*

♥ North Country Glycerine Soap ■
7888 County Rd. #6
Maple Plain, MN 55359-9552
(800)328-4827, (612)479-3381
Personal care, Companion animal

♥ North Pacific Naturals ✳ ■
24855 W. Brush Creek Rd.
Sweet Home, OR 97386-9614
(800)882-9887, (541)367-8629
Personal care

◆ Northern Labs, Inc. ✳ ■
P.O. Box 850
Manitowoc, WI 54221
(920)684-7137
Personal care

◆ No-Tweeze
(see Kenra, Inc.)

◆ NOW® Products, Inc. ✳ ■
P.O. Box 27608
Tempe, AZ 85285-7608
(800)662-0333, (602)966-6100
Household

▼ Noxell Corp. ■
200 Park Ave.
New York, NY 10166
(212)682-0883
(see parent Procter & Gamble)
Personal care

▼ Noxema
(see Procter & Gamble)

♥ Nu Skin International, Inc. ■
75 W. Center St.
Provo, UT 84601
(800)877-6100, (801)345-1000
Personal care

♥ Nuhairtrition
(see Hobe Laboratories, Inc.)

◆ Nutra Nail
(see CCA Industries, Inc.)

♥ Nutraceutical Corp. ■
1500 Kearns Blvd, Ste. B200
Park City, UT 84060-7330
(800)373-9660, (801)655-6001
Personal care

◆ Nutribiotic ■
133 Copeland St., Ste. C
Petaluma, CA 94952-3181
(707)769-2266
Personal care, Household

♥ Nutri-Cell, Inc. ■
1038 N. Tustin, Ste. 309
Orange, CA 92667-5958
(714)953-8307
Personal care, Cosmetics

◆ Nu-Trish'N
(see Aloette Cosmetics, Inc.)

▼ o.b. Tampons
(see Personal Products Co.)

▼ Obsession
(see Calvin Klein Cosmetics Co.)

▼ O-Cel-O™
(see 3M™)

◆ Odomaster
(see Surco Products, Inc.)

◆ Odor-B-Gone Products
(see Gannon's, Inc.)

▼ OFF! Products
(see S.C. Johnson & Son, Inc.)

▼ Ogilvie
(see Playtex Products, Inc.)

❤ Ohio Hempery ■ ● ⊠
7002 St., Route 329
Guysville, OH 45735
(800)BUY-HEMP, (614)662-4367
Personal care

▼ Oil of Olay
(see Procter & Gamble)

◆ Oil-Dri Corporation
of America ✳ ■ ●
410 N. Michigan Ave., Ste. 400
Chicago, IL 60611
(800)634-0315, (312)321-1515
Companion animal

▼ Old English
(see Reckitt & Colman)

▼ Old Spice
(see Procter & Gamble)

❤ Oliva Stuard
(see Natural Bodycare)

▼ One Touch
(see Johnson & Johnson)

❤ One UnLimited Perfume
(see LPI, Inc.)

❤ OPI Products, Inc. ■
13056 Saticoy St.
N. Hollywood, CA 91605
(800)341-9999, (818)759-2400
Personal care, Cosmetics

◆ Optikem Int'l, Inc. ✳ ■
P.O. Box 27319
Denver, CO 80227
(303)936-1137
Personal care

◆ Optimum
(see Lobob Laboratories, Inc.)

◆ Optisoap
(see Optikem Int'l, Inc.)

◆ Orajel
(see Del Laboratories, Inc.)

❤ Oral-B
(see Gillette Co.)

◆ Orange-Mate Inc. ✳ ■
P.O. Box 883
Waldport, OR 97394
(800)626-8685
Household

❤ Orange-Plus® Cleaner
(see Earth Friendly Products)

▼ Orchard Mist
(see Melaleuca)

◆ Oregon Soap, Co. ■
P.O. Box 14464
Portland, OR 97293-0464
(800)549-0299
Personal care

◆ Organic Aid Products
(see Buty-Wave Products Co., Inc.)

❤ Organic Essentials ✳ ■
822 Baldridge St.
O'Donnell, TX 79351
(800)765-6491, (806)428-3486
Personal care

❤ Origins Skin Care Products
(see Estee Lauder Companies)

❤ Orlane, Inc. ■ ●
555 Madison Ave., 20th Fl.
New York, NY 10022
(212)750-1111
Cosmetics

❤ Orly International, Inc. ■
9309 Deering Ave.
Chatsworth, CA 91311
(818)998-1111
Cosmetics

◆ Otto Basics-Beauty 2 Go! ✳ ■
P.O. Box 9023
Rancho Sante Fe, CA 92067
(800)598-OTTO
Cosmetics

❤ Outrageous™
(see Revlon, Inc.)

◆ Oxford
(see Essette Corp.)

▼ Oxydol
(see Procter & Gamble)

♥ Oxyfresh Worldwide, Inc. ●
East 12928 Indiana Ave.
Spokane, WA 99216-4999
(509)924-4999
Personal care, Household,
Companion animal

▼ P.O.M. Hair Products
(see Luster Products, Inc.)

◆ Pacific Coast
(see Surco Products, Inc.)

◆ Pad Guard
(see Trophy Animal Health Care)

▼ Palm Beach Beauty Products ■
950 Xenia Ave. S.
Minneapolis, MN 55416
(800)326-7256, (612)546-0322
Personal care, Cosmetics,
Household, Companion animal

▼ Palmolive
(see Colgate-Palmolive Co.)

◆ Paloma Picasso Fragrances
(see L'Oreal of Paris)

▼ Pampers
(see Procter & Gamble)

▼ Pantene
(see Procter & Gamble)

◆ Papaya Enzyme Mask
(see MW Laboratories)

♥ Papaya Pineapple Enzyme
Peel & Mask
(see Jason Natural Products)

♥ Para Laboratories, Inc. ■
100 Rose Ave.
Hempstead, NY 11550
(800)645-3752, (516)538-4600
Personal care

◆ Parfums Cacharel & Cie. ■
6 Rue Graviers, F-92521
Neuilly-sur-Seine, France
01-46-40-5814
(see parent L'Oreal of Paris)
Cosmetics

▼ Parfums International Ltd.
(see Unilever United States Inc.)

♥ Parker
(see Gillette Co.)

◆ Parlux Fragrances, Inc. ✳ ■ ●
3725 S.W. 30th Ave.
Fort Lauderdale, FL 33312
(954)316-9008
Personal care

▼ Parson's Ammonia
(see Church & Dwight Co., Inc.)

▼ Passion
(see Elizabeth Arden Co.)

◆ Passionflower Massage Oil
(see Tropical Botanicals)

◆ Patricia Allison ■ ● ✉
4470 Monahan Rd.
La Mesa, CA 91941
(800)858-8742, (619)444-4879
Personal care, Cosmetics

❤ Paul Mitchell Products
(see John Paul Mitchell Systems)

◆ Paul Penders Co., Inc. ■
1340 Commerce St.
Petaluma, CA 94954
(800)440-7285, (707)763-5828
Personal care, Cosmetics

❤ Paula's Choice—Beginning
Press ✳ ● ✉
13075 Gateway Dr., #300
Tukwila, WA 98168-3342
(800)831-4088
Personal care, Cosmetics

◆ P-Bee Products ■ ●
8280 -123 Clairemont Mesa Blvd.
San Diego, CA 92111
(619)560-7945
Personal care, Cosmetics

▼ PCJ Hair Products
(see Luster Products, Inc.)

❤ Peelu ✳ ■
109 1/2 Broadway
Fargo, ND 58102
(701)281-0511
Personal care

◆ Pendaflex
(see Essette Corp.)

❤ Penn Herb Co., Ltd. ■ ● ✉
10601 Decatur Rd., Ste. 3
Philadelphia, PA 19154-3293
(215)925-3336
Personal care

- ❤ Penny Island Products ■
  P.O.Box 521
  Graton, CA 95444-0521
  (707)823-2406
  Personal care

- ▼ Pepsodent
  (see Chesebrough-Pond's USA Co.)

- ❤ Perfect Balance Skincare Products
  (see Marilyn Miglin L.P.)

- ◆ Performance Plus
  (see Aloette Cosmetics, Inc.)

- ▼ Performaxx
  (see Clorox Company)

- ❤ Perfumoils, Inc. dba Homebody ●
  P.O. Box 2266
  W. Brattleboro, VT 05303
  (802)254-6280
  Personal care

- ❤ Perlier Natural Recipes
  (see LPI, Inc.)

- ◆ Perm Repair
  (see Pro-Line Corp.)

- ◆ Permathene 12
  (see CCA Industries, Inc.)

- ▼ Peroxicare® Toothpaste
  (see Church & Dwight Co., Inc.)

- ◆ Perry Ellis Fragrances
  (see Parlux Fragrances, Inc.)

- ❤ Person & Covey ✳ ■
  616 Allen Ave.
  Glendale, CA 91201
  (818)240-1030
  Personal care

- ▼ Personal Products Co. ■
  199 Grandview Rd.
  Skillman, NJ 08558-9418
  (see parent Johnson & Johnson)
  Personal care

- ❤ Personna®
  (see American Safety Razor Co.)

- ▼ Pert Plus
  (see Procter & Gamble)

- ❤ Pet Air®
  (see Mia Rose Products)

- ❤ Pet Organics
  (see Baxter Environmental
  Products)

- ◆ Pet Pillars
  (see Trophy Animal Health Care)

109

♥ PetGuard, Inc. ✳ ■
165 Industrial Loop S., Unit #5
Orange Park, FL 32073
(800)874-3221
Companion animal

♥ Petrelief Products
(see St. JON Laboratories)

♥ Petrodex
(see St. JON Laboratories)

♥ Petromalt
(see St. JON Laboratories)

♥ Pharmagel Corp. ✳ ■
P.O. Box 2288
Monterey, CA 93942-2288
(800)882-4889, (805)568-0022
Personal care, Cosmetics

♥ Pheromone
(see Marilyn Miglin L.P.)

♥ Philip B. Hair &
Body Care ✳ ■ ● ✉
P.O. Box 15341
Beverly Hills, CA 90209
(800)643-5556
Cosmetics

◆ Philosophy
(see BioMedic Clinical Care)

♥ Phybiosis ✳ ●
P.O. Box 992
Bowie, MD 20718
(301)805-7920
Personal care

◆ Physically Handicapped,
Inc. ✳ ■ ✉
4002 Minden Ave.
Texarkana, AR 71854
(870)773-4901
Household, Companion animal

◆ Phyto Care
(see Dr. Grandel)

♥ Pickering & Simmons, LLC ✉
2031 Route 130, Ste. D
Monmouth Junction, NJ 08852
Personal care

◆ Pilot Corp. of America ■
60 Commerce Dr.
Trumbull, CT 06611
(203)377-8800
Household

◆ Pine Glo Products, Inc. ✳ ■
P.O. Box 429, Hwy. 401
Rolesville, NC 27571
(919)556-7787
Household

▼ Pine Sol
(see Clorox Company)

▼ Pink Oil Moisturizer Lotion
(see Luster Products, Inc.)

◆ Planet Inc. ✳ ■
P.O. Box 48184, 3575 Douglas St.
Victoria, BC, V8Z 7H6, Canada
(800)858-8449, (250)478-8171
Household

❤ Plant Therapy®
(see Mia Rose Products)

▼ Playtex Products, Inc. ■
300 Nyala Farms Rd.
Westport, CT 06880
(203)341-4000
Personal care, Household

▼ Playtex® Tampons
(see Playtex Products, Inc.)

❤ Pleasures
(see Estee Lauder Companies)

▼ Pledge
(see S.C. Johnson & Son, Inc.)

◆ Plus-White Toothpaste
(see CCA Industries, Inc.)

▼ Poise
(see Kimberly-Clark Corp.)

▼ Polident® Denture Cleaner
(see Block Drug Co.)

◆ Polo by Ralph Lauren
(see L'Oreal of Paris)

▼ Ponds
(see Chesebrough-Pond's USA Co.)

▼ Post-It® Notes
(see 3M™)

◆ Post-Op
(see MW Laboratories)

❤ Poudre Lumiere
(see La Prairie, Inc.)

◆ Power Plus
(see Granny's Old
Fashioned Products)

▼ Power Stick
(see Chesebrough-Pond's USA Co.)

◆ Prairie Meadows Herbal
Soap Co. ✳ ■ ● ✉
P.O. Box 292356
Phelan, CA 92329
(760)868-4350
Personal care

- Precious Collection
  Aromatherapy * ■ ● ▫
  P.O. Box 17155
  Boulder, CO 80308
  (800)877-6889, (303)447-1667
  Personal care

- Preference
  (see L'Oreal of Paris)

- Prell
  (see Procter & Gamble)

- Premier One Products
  (see Nutraceutical Corp.)

- Prescription Diet
  (see Hill's Pet Nutrition)

- Prescriptives Treatment &
  Cosmetic Products
  (see Estee Lauder Companies)

- Pretty Please
  (see Change of Face Cosmetics)

- Prima Fleur Botanicals, Inc. ■
  1525 E. Francisco Blvd., Ste. 16
  San Rafael, CA 94901
  (415)455-0957
  Personal care, Cosmetics

- Prince Matchabelli
  (see Chesebrough-Pond's USA Co.)

- Princess Livia
  (see Cosmetique, Inc.)

- Princess Marcella Borghese, Inc. ■
  767 Fifth Ave.
  New York, NY 10153
  (212)572-5000
  (see parent Revlon, Inc.)
  Cosmetics

- Pro-Care
  (see Melaleuca)

- Procter & Gamble Co. ■
  One Procter & Gamble Plaza
  Cincinnati, OH 45201
  (800)543-1745
  *Personal care, Cosmetics,
  Household, Companion animal*

- Professional Pet Products * ■
  1873 NW 97th Ave.
  Miami, FL 33172
  (800)432-5349, (305)592-1992
  Companion animal

- Professional®
  (see Home Service Products Co.)

- PROFILE
  (see Flowery Beauty Products)

◆ Pro-Line Corp. ■ ●
P.O. Box 223706
Dallas, TX 75222
(800)527-5879, (214)631-4247
Personal care

◆ Pro-Perm
(see CCA Industries, Inc.)

◆ Propha pH
(see Del Laboratories, Inc.)

◆ Pro-Tec Pet Health ■ ●
5440 Camus Rd.
Carson City, NV 89701-9306
(800)44-FLEAS, (510)676-9600
Companion animal

◆ Protect®
(see John O. Butler Co.)

▼ Protein 21 Shampoo & Hairspray
(see Mennen Co.)

▼ Protein 29 Hair Groom
(see Mennen Co.)

❤ Provence Santé
(see Baudelaire, Inc.)

❤ Psoria-Gard
(see Hobe Laboratories, Inc.)

▼ Puffs
(see Procter & Gamble)

▼ Pull-Ups®
(see Kimberly-Clark Corp.)

❤ Pure & Basic Products
(see Neo Tech Cosmetic, Inc.)

❤ Pure & Natural® Soap
(see Dial Corporation)

❤ Pure Essentials®
(see Earth Science, Inc.)

❤ Pure Touch Therapeutics ✳ ■ ●
P.O. Box 2234
Glen Ellen, CA 95442-0234
(800)442-PURE, (707)996-7817
Personal care

❤ Purex®
(see Dial Corporation)

▼ Purex Toss N' Soft
(see Church & Dwight Co., Inc.)

❤ Purifiles
(see Flowery Beauty Products)

▼ Purpose Moisturizer
(see Johnson & Johnson)

◆ Pyrethi-Care
(see Espree Animal Products, Inc.)

▼ Q-Tips Products
(see Chesebrough-Pond's USA Co.)

▼ Quantum
(see Helene Curtis Int'l)

❤ Queen Helene
(see Para Laboratories, Inc.)

◆ Quencher Cosmetics ■
565 Broad Hollow Rd.
Farmingdale, NY 11735
(516)293-7070
(see parent Del Laboratories, Inc.)
Cosmetics

❤ Quinta Essentia
(see Norimoor, Inc.)

❤ Rachel Perry, Inc. ✳ ●
9800 Eton Ave.
Chatsworth, CA 91311-4307
(800)966-8888
Personal care, Cosmetics

▼ Raid
(see S.C. Johnson & Son, Inc.)

▼ Rain Drops
(see Church & Dwight Co., Inc.)

❧ Rainbath
(see Neutrogena Corp.)

❤ Rainbow Products
(see Rainbow Research Corp.)

❤ Rainbow Research Corp. ■ ⊠
170 Wilbur Pl.
Bohemia, NY 11716
(800)722-9595, (516)589-5563
Personal care

◆ Rainforest Body Wash
(see Tropical Botanicals)

❤ Rainforest Co. ✳ ■ ⊠
141 Millwell Dr.
Maryland Heights, MO 63043
(314)344-1000
Personal care

❤ Rainforest®
(see Rachel Perry, Inc)

❤ Rain-X
(see Unelko Corp.)

◆ Ralph Lauren Fragrance Division ■
575 Fifth Ave.
New York, NY 10017
(212)818-1500
(see parent L'Oreal of Paris)
Cosmetics

▼ Rave
(see Chesebrough Pond's USA Co.)

❤ Ravenwood ✳ ◼
5110 M-72 W.
Traverse City, MI 49684
(616)929-4181
Personal care

❤ Ravenwood Essential Oils
(see Borlind of Germany)

❤ Real Aloe Co. ◼
P.O. Box 2770
Oxnard, CA 93033
(800)541-7809
Personal care

❤ Real Goods Trading Corp. ▣
200 Clara Ave.
Ukiah, CA 95482-4004
(707)468-9292
Personal care, Household

❤ Real Natural Products ◼
P.O. Box 10761
Pompano Beach, FL 33061
(800)653-4006
(see parent TCCD Int'l)
Cosmetics

❤ Really Works
(see Vin-Dotco, Inc.)

▼ Reckitt & Colman Inc. ◼
1800 Valley Rd.
Wayne, NJ 07470
(973)686-0279
Household

▼ Red Door Fragrance
(see Elizabeth Arden Co.)

▼ Red Fragrance
(see Procter & Gamble)

◆ Redken Labs, Inc. ◼
575 Fifth Ave.
New York, NY 10017
(212)818-1500
(see parent L'Oreal of Paris)
Personal care

❤ Redmond Minerals, Inc. ✳ ◼
6005 North 100 West
Redmond, UT 84652
(800)367-7258, (435)529-7486
*Personal care, Household,
Companion animal*

❦ Redmond Products, Inc. ◼
18930 W. 78th St.
Chanhassen, MN 55317
(612)934-4868
(see parent Bristol-Myers Squibb Co.)
Personal care

◆ Refresh All Purpose Cleaner
(see Pine Glo Products, Inc.)

◆ Rejuveniss
(see Dreamous Corp.)

◆ Rejuvia Vitamin E Skin
Care Products ■
565 Broad Hollow Rd.
Farmingdale, NY 11735
(516)293-7070
(see parent Del Laboratories, Inc.)
Personal care

◆ Rembrandt Toothpaste &
Mouthwash
(see Den-Mat Corp.)

❤ Remington Products Co., L.L.C. ✳ ■
60 Main St.
Bridgeport, CT 06604
(800)736-4648
Personal care

◆ Renew Carpet Cleaner
(see Pine Glo Products, Inc.)

▼ ReNu® Solution
(see Bausch & Lomb Inc.)

❤ Renuzit®
(see Dial Corporation)

▼ Resolve
(see Reckitt & Colman)

❤ Resplenda
(see Vanda Beauty Counselors, Inc.)

❤ Res-Q-Dent Sensitivity Pain Relief
(see Eco-Dent Int'l, Inc.)

◆ Restor Products
(see Buty-Wave Products Co., Inc.)

❤ Reviva Labs, Inc. ■
705 Hopkins Rd.
Haddonfield, NJ 08033
(800)257-7774, (609)428-3885
Personal care, Cosmetics

❤ Revlon Perfect Finish Razors
(see American Safety Razor Co.)

❤ Revlon, Inc. ■
625 Madison Ave.
New York, NY 10022
(800)4Revlon, (212)527-4000
Personal care, Cosmetics

❤ Rexall Showcase Int'l ■ ● ⬚
851 Broken Sound Pkwy., NW
Boca Raton, FL 33487
(800)327-0908, (561)241-9400
Personal care, Cosmetics

▼ Rhuli Products
(see S.C. Johnson & Son, Inc.)

◆ Rich & Radiant
(see Granny's Old Fashioned
Products)

▼ Richardson-Vicks, Inc. ■
One Procter & Gamble Plaza
Cincinnati, OH 45202
(513)983-1100
(see parent Procter & Gamble)
Personal care

❤ Right Guard
(see Gillette Co.)

▼ Rinso
(see Lever Brothers)

❤ Rivers Run ✳ ●
25261 Calle Busca
Lake Forest, CA 92630-2604
(310)545-8933
Household

▼ Roach Motel
(see Clorox Company)

❤ Roebic Laboratories, Inc. ✳ ■
25 Connair Rd., P.O. Box 927
Orange, CT 06477
(203)795-1283
Household

❤ Roffler & Framesi Hair Care
(see Framesi USA/Roffler)

❤ Rosemary Foot Balsam
(see Dr. Hauschka
Cosmetics USA Inc.)

◆ Rotex
(see Essette Corp.)

❤ Royal Jelly Conditioner
(see Nutraceutical Corp.)

❤ Russ Kalvin Hair Care
(see Allon Personal Care Corp.)

▼ S.C. Johnson & Son, Inc. ■
1525 Howe St.
Racine, WI 53403-2236
(800)558-5252, (414)260-2000
Household

▼ S.O.S.
(see Clorox Company)

◆ SA8® Laundry Detergents
(see Amway Corp.)

◆ Sacred Sage
(see Medicine Flower)

◆ Safari by Ralph Lauren
(see L'Oreal of Paris)

- ❤ Safe Choice®
  (see American Formulating &
  Manufacturing)

- ❤ Safe Solutions, Inc. ✳ ■
  10265 Miller Rd., #102
  Dallas, TX 75238-1224
  (877)554-5222, (214)221-5222
  Personal care, Companion animal

- ▼ Safeguard
  (see Procter & Gamble)

- ◆ SaFur
  (see Physically Handicapped, Inc.)

- ◆ Sally Hansen Cosmetics ■
  178 EAB Plaza
  Uniondale, NY 11556
  (516)844-2020
  (see parent Del Laboratories, Inc.)
  Personal care, Cosmetics

- ◆ Salon Naturals
  (see ShiKai Products)

- ▼ Salon Selectives
  (see Helene Curtis Int'l)

- ▼ Sani-Flush
  (see Reckitt & Colman)

- ❤ Sante
  (see Logona USA, Inc.)

- ❤ Sappo Hill Soapworks ✳ ■
  654 Tolman Creek Rd.
  Ashland, OR 97520
  (541)482-4485
  Personal care

- ❤ Sara St. James
  (see Cosmetique, Inc.)

- ❤ Sarah Michaels, Inc. ■
  180 Campanelli Pkwy.
  Stoughton, MA 02072
  (800)527-2869, (781)341-8810
  (see parent Dial Corporation)
  Personal care

- ❤ Sarakan
  (see Baudelaire, Inc.)

- ▼ Saran Wrap
  (see S.C. Johnson & Son, Inc.)

- ❤ Satin Care
  (see Gillette Co.)

- ❤ Satin Floss
  (see Gillette Co.)

- ▼ Schick
  (see Warner-Lambert Co.)

❤ Schwarzkopf & Dep Inc. ■ ⊠
2101 E. Via Arado Ave.
Rancho Dominguez, CA 90220
(800)367-2855, (310)604-0777
Personal care

▼ Science Diet
(see Hill's Pet Nutrition)

▼ Scoop Away
(see Clorox Company)

▼ Scope
(see Procter & Gamble)

▼ Scotch™ Magic™ Tape
(see 3M™)

▼ Scotch-Brite™
(see 3M™)

▼ Scotchgard™
(see 3M™)

▼ Scott Paper Co.
(see Kimberly-Clark Corp.)

◆ Scotties
(see Irving Tissue, Inc.)

◆ Scrubb 'N Sluff
(see Aloette Cosmetics, Inc.)

▼ Scrubbing Bubbles
(see S.C. Johnson & Son, Inc.)

❤ Scruples Professional Salon
Products, Inc. ✳ ■ ●
8231-214th St., West
Lakeville, MN 55044-9102
(612)469-4646
Personal care

▼ S-Curl Hair Products
(see Luster Products, Inc.)

➤ Sea Breeze
(see Cairol, Inc.)

❤ Sea Minerals Co. ✳ ■ ●
2886 Heath Ave.
Bronx, NY 10463-7847
(718)796-5509
Personal care, Cosmetics

❤ Sebastian Int'l, Inc. ●
6109 DeSoto Ave.
Woodland Hills, CA 91367
(800)829-7322, (818)999-5112
Personal care, Cosmetics

▼ Secret
(see Procter & Gamble)

119

♥ Secret Gardens ✳ ■ ● ⊠
P.O. Box B
Fall Creek, OR 97438
(800)537-8766
Personal care

▼ Security Tampons
(see Kimberly-Clark Corp.)

♥ Seide® Hair Care
(see Borlind of Germany)

◆ Sensitive Balance
(see Dr. Grandel)

▼ Sensitive Eyes® Solution
(see Bausch & Lomb Inc.)

▼ Sensodyne®
(see Block Drug Co.)

♥ Sensor Products
(see Gillette Co.)

◆ Sereine Cleaning Solution
(see Optikem Int'l, Inc.)

▼ Serene
(see Melaleuca)

◆ SerVaas Laboratories Inc. ✳ ■
1200 Waterway Blvd.
Indianapolis, IN 46207
(800)433-5818, (317)636-7760
Household

▼ Sesame St. Children's Bath Products
(see Softsoap Enterprises)

♥ Set-N-Me-Free Aloe Vera Co. ■
19220 SE Stark
Portland, OR 97233-5751
(800)221-9727, (503)666-9661
*Personal care, Cosmetics,
Companion animal*

♥ Seventh Generation ✳ ■
1 Mill St.
Burlington, VT 05446
(802)658-3773
Household

♥ Shadow Lake, Inc. ✳ ■
P.O. Box 2597
Danbury, CT 06813-2597
(800)343-6588, (203)778-0881
Personal care, Household

♥ Shaklee Corp. ■ ●
4747 Willow Dr.
Pleasanton, CA 94080
(800)SHAKLEE, (925)924-2000
*Personal care, Cosmetics,
Household*

◆ Shamana
(see Medicine Flower)

▼ Shield
(see Lever Brothers)

❤ ShiKai Products ■
P.O. Box 2866
Santa Rosa, CA 95405
(800)448-0298
Personal care

◆ Shivani Ayurvedic
(see Devi, Inc.)

▼ Shout
(see S.C. Johnson & Son, Inc.)

❤ Shower 2000
(see Bonne Bell, Inc.)

▼ Shower Shine
(see S.C. Johnson & Son, Inc.)

▼ Shower to Shower
(see Johnson & Johnson)

❤ Siddha Int'l ✳ ■
P.O. Box 5127
Gainesville, FL 32605
(904)376-8173
Personal care, Cosmetics

❤ Sierra Dawn Products ✳ ■
P.O. Box 1203
Sebastopol, CA 95472
(707)588-0755
Personal care, Household

▼ Signal Mouthwash
(see Chesebrough-Pond's USA Co.)

❤ Silkience
(see Gillette Co.)

❤ Simmons Natural Bodycare ■ ▣
42295 Hwy. 36
Bridgeville, CA 95526-9603
(707)777-1920
*Personal care, Household,
Companion animal*

◆ Simple Green
(see Sunshine Makers, Inc.)

❤ Simpler Thyme® ■ ▣
P.O. Box 2858
Branchville, NJ 07826
(973)875-9070
Personal care

❤ Simplers Botanical Co. ✳ ■
P.O. Box 39
Forestville, CA 95436
(707)887-2012
Personal care

❤ Simply Bath
(see Arizona Natural Resources, Inc.)

❤ Sinclair & Valentine
(see Smith & Vandiver)

❤ Sistina
(see Cosmetique, Inc.)

❤ Skeeter Skatter™
(see Simmons Natural Bodycare)

▼ Skin Bracer
(see Mennen Co.)

❤ Skin Caviar
(see La Prairie, Inc.)

◆ Skin Med
(see MW Laboratories)

◆ Skin Savvy
(see Strong Skin Savvy)

❤ Skin Trip
(see Mountain Ocean)

❤ Skin Zyme
(see Beauty Naturally, Inc.)

❤ Skinovations®
(see Rachel Perry, Inc)

❤ Skin-So-Soft
(see Avon Products, Inc.)

▼ Skintimate Shaving Products
(see S.C. Johnson & Son, Inc.)

❤ Smackers
(see Bonne Bell, Inc.)

❤ Smith & Vandiver, Inc. ■
480 Airport Blvd.
Watsonville, CA 95076
(831)722-9526
Personal care

▼ SmithKline Beecham
Consumer Healthcare ■
100 Beecham Dr.
Pittsburgh, PA 15205
(800)456-6670, (412)928-1000
Personal care

◆ SNAP All Purpose Cleaner
(see Pine Glo Products, Inc.)

▼ Sno Bowl Toilet Bowl Cleaner
(see Church & Dwight Co., Inc.)

▼ Sno Drops
(see Church & Dwight Co., Inc.)

▼ Snowy
(see Reckitt & Colman)

▼ Snuggle
(see Lever Brothers)

❤ Soap Factory ■ ●
141 Cushman Rd.
St. Catherines, Ontario, L2M 6T2
Canada
Personal care, Household

❤ Soap Works ■ ●
883 Lake Drive N
Keswick, Ontario L4P 3E9
Canada
(416)489-8016
Personal care, Household,
Companion animal

◆ Sof/Pro Clean
(see Lobob Laboratories, Inc.)

◆ Soft & Beautiful
(see Pro-Line Corp.)

❤ Soft & Dri
(see Gillette Co.)

▼ Soft Scrub
(see Clorox Company)

▼ Softsoap Enterprises ■
134 Columbia St. South
Chaska, MN 55318
(612-)448-4799
(see parent Colgate-Palmolive Co.)
Personal care, Household

▼ Softsoap Liquid Soap Products
(see Softsoap Enterprises)

◆ Softweve
(see Irving Tissue, Inc.)

◆ Soil Away
(see Granny's Old Fashioned
Products)

◆ Soilove Laundry Soil &
Stain Remover
(see America's Finest Products Corp.)

❤ Sojourner Farms ✳ ■
1 19th Ave. South
Minneapolis, MN 55454-1021
(888)867-6567
Companion animal

❤ Solid Gold Health Products
for Pets, Inc. ■ ▨
1483 N. Cuyamaca
El Cajon, CA 92020
(619)258-2780
Companion animal

❤ Solo Para Ti Cosmetics
(see AM Cosmetics, Inc.)

123

◆ Solor Cosmetic Labs, Inc. ✳ ■
4920 NW 165th St.
Miami, FL 33014
(800)327-3991, (305)621-5551
Personal care, Cosmetics

❤ Sombra Cosmetics Inc. ✳ ■ ▣
5600 - G McLeod, NE
Albuquerque, NM 87109
(800)225-3963, (505)888-0288
Cosmetics

◆ Song of Life ■ ▣
P.O. Box 294
Rock Cave, WV 26234
(304)924-5839
Personal care, Companion animal

❤ Sonoma Soap Co.
(see Avalon Natural Products)

◆ Soothing Touch
(see Sunshine)

▼ Sothy's USA ■ ●
1500 N.W. 94th Ave.
Miami, FL 33172
(800)325-0503
Personal care, Cosmetics

❤ Spa Essentials
(see Earth Science, Inc.)

◆ Sparkle Glass Cleaner
(see A.J. Funk & Co.)

◆ Sparkle Paper Products
(see Georgia Pacific Corp.)

◆ Specialty Products, Inc. ✳ ■
10300 Farm Rd. 1902
Crowley, TX 76036
(800)860-1615
Household, Companion animal

▼ Speed Stick
(see Mennen Co.)

❤ Spellbound
(see Estee Lauder Companies)

▼ Spic & Span
(see Procter & Gamble)

❤ Spirit Stones
(see Siddha Int'l)

▼ Splendor
(see Elizabeth Arden Co.)

▼ Spray 'n Wash
(see Reckitt & Colman)

♥ St. Clair Industries, Inc. ✳ ■
3067 E. Commercial Blvd.
Ft. Lauderdale, FL 33308
(954)491-0400
Personal care, Companion animal

🦴 St. Ives Laboratories ■
2525 Armitage Ave.
Melrose Park, IL 60160
(708)450-3000
(see parent Alberto-Culver Co.)
Personal care

♥ St. John's Herb
Garden, Inc. ✳ ■ ● ⊠
7711 Hillmeade Rd.
Bowie, MD 20720
(301)262-5302
Personal care

♥ St. JON Laboratories ■
1656 West 240th St.
Harbor City, CA 90710
(800)969-7387, (310)326-2720
Companion animal

♥ St. JON Naturals
(see St. JON Laboratories)

♥ StaFlo® Starch
(see Dial Corporation)

◆ Stain Blaster Products
(see Specialty Products, Inc.)

▼ Stain Out
(see Clorox Company)

◆ Star Brite ✳ ■
4041 S.W. 47th Ave.
Fort Lauderdale, FL 33314
(800)327-8583, (305)587-6280
Household

♥ Star of the East Incence
(see Secret Gardens)

♥ Starwest Botanicals, Inc. ■
11253 Trade Center Dr.
Rancho Cordova, CA 95742
(800)800-4372, (916)853-9354
Personal care

▼ Static Guard
(see Alberto-Culver Co.)

▼ Stayfree
(see Personal Products Co.)

▼ Step Saver
(see S.C. Johnson & Son, Inc.)

♥ Steps In Health, Ltd. ⊠
P.O. Box 604426
Bayside, NY 11360-4426
(800)471-VEGE, (516)471-2432
Personal care

♥ Sterling Clean ✳ ■
P.O. Box 20016
Austin, TX 78720-0126
(512)445-7940
Household

▼ Stick-Ups
(see Reckitt & Colman)

◆ Stick-With-Us Products, Inc. ✳ ■
#4-1151 Horse Shoe Way
Richmond, BC, V7A 4S5
Canada
(800)492-9464, (604)241-0448
Personal care

♥ Stonybrook Botanicals
(see Rainbow Research Corp.)

▼ STP Corporation ■
83 Wooster Heights Rd., Bldg. 301
Danbury, CT 06813
(203)731-2300
(see parent Clorox Company)
Household

◆ Straight Arrow Products ■ ⊠
P.O. Box 20350
Lehigh Valley, PA 18002
(800)736-5155
Personal care

♥ Streetwear
(see Revlon, Inc.)

◆ Stress-A-Dine
(see Trophy Animal Health Care)

◆ Strong Skin Savvy, Inc. ■
1 Lakeside Dr.
New Providence, PA 17560
(800)724-3952, (717)786-8947
Personal care

◆ Studio Line Hair
(see L'Oreal of Paris)

♥ Studio Magic, Inc. ✳ ● ⊠
20135-Cypress Creek Dr.
Alva, FL 33920-3305
(941)728-3344
Personal care, Cosmetics

♥ Styling Technology Corp. ■ ●
7400 E. Tierra Buena Ln.
Scottsdale, AZ 85260
(480)609-6000
Personal care, Cosmetics

▼ Suave
(see Helene Curtis Int'l)

◆ Sudden Change
(see CCA Industries, Inc.)

◆ Sue's Amazing Lip Stuff ■
P.O. Box 64
Westby, WI 54667
608-634-2988
Personal care, Cosmetics

❤ Sukésha
(see Chuckles, Inc.)

❤ Sul Ray
(see Alvin Last, Inc.)

❤ Sumeru Garden Herbals ✳ ■
P.O. Box 325
Twin Lakes, WI 53181
(800)478-6378
Personal care

◆ Sun and Earth Products
(see McWolf Enterprises)

◆ Sun Dog Products
(see Sue's Amazing Lip Stuff)

▼ Sun Shades
(see Melaleuca)

❤ Sun Smackers
(see Bonne Bell, Inc.)

❤ Sunaturals
(see Hobe Laboratories, Inc.)

▼ Sundown Sunscreen
(see Johnson & Johnson)

❤ Sunfeather Natural Soap Co. ■ ✉
1551 Hwy. 72
Potsdam, NY 13676
(315)265-3648
Personal care, Companion animal

▼ Sunflowers
(see Elizabeth Arden Co.)

▼ Sunlight
(see Lever Brothers)

❤ Sunlind
(see Borlind of Germany)

◆ Sunsect
(see Amon-Re Laboratories)

◆ Sunshine ✳ ■
1616 Preuss Rd.
Los Angeles, CA 90035
(800)225-3623
Personal care

◆ Sunshine Makers, Inc. ■
P.O. Box 2708
Huntington Beach, CA 92647
(800)228-0709
Household

❤ SunSwat
(see Kiss My Face Corp.)

◆ Super Cell Liquid
(see Trophy Animal Health Care)

❤ Supernail ■
2220 Gaspar Ave.
City of Commerce, CA 90040
(323)728-2999
(see parent American Int'l Ind.)
Personal care, Cosmetics

▼ Supreme Steel Wool
(see Church & Dwight Co., Inc.)

◆ Surco Products, Inc. ✳ ■
RIDC Industrial Park
292 Alpha Dr.
Pittsburgh, PA 15238-2903
(800)556-0111, (412)252-7000
Household

◆ Surcotech
(see Surco Products, Inc.)

▼ Sure
(see Procter & Gamble)

▼ Sure & Natural
(see Personal Products Co.)

◆ Sure Grow 100
(see Trophy Animal Health Care)

▼ Surf
(see Lever Brothers)

❤ Surrey, Inc. ■
13110 Trails End Rd.
Leander, TX 78641
(512)267-7172
Personal care

❤ Swan Lake Botanicals ■ ▣
612 Dockery Lane
Mineral Bluff, GA 30559-2701
(706)492-9927
*Personal care, Cosmetics,
Companion animal*

❤ Swedish Clover
(see Flowery Beauty Products)

❤ Sweet Georgia Brown
Cosmetics & Hair Care
(see AM Cosmetics, Inc.)

▼ Swiffer Products
(see Procter & Gamble)

꩜ Swiss Formula Products
(see St. Ives Laboratories)

❤ Swy Flotter
(see Kiss My Face Corp.)

❤ T-Tree®
(see Earth Science, Inc.)

❤ T.N. Dickinson ✻ ●
31 E. High St.
East Hampton, CT 06424
(888)860-2279, (860)267-2279
Personal care, Cosmetics

꩜ T/Gel®
(see Neutrogena Corp.)

꩜ T/Scalp®
(see Neutrogena Corp.)

▼ Tambrands, Inc. ■
P.O. Box 599
Cincinnati, OH 45273
(800)523-0014, (513)983-1100
(see parent Procter & Gamble)
Personal care

❤ Tame
(see Gillette Co.)

▼ Tampax Tampons
(see Tambrands, Inc.)

▼ Tanner's Preserve
(see Clorox Company)

◆ Tanning Research Labs, Inc. ✻ ■
Box 265111
Daytona Beach, FL 32126
(904)677-9559
Personal care, Cosmetics

▼ Targon® Smokers' Mouthwash
(see Block Drug Co.)

▼ Tarni-Shield™ Fine
Metal Polishes
(see 3M™)

❤ TARRAH ✻ ●
1501 Northpoint Pkwy., Ste. 100
West Palm Beach, FL 33407
(561)640-5700
Personal care, Cosmetics

❤ TaUT by Leonard
Engelman ■ ● ⊠
9428 Eton, Ste. M
Chatsworth, CA 91311
(800)438-8288, (818)773-3975
Personal care, Cosmetics

129

▼ TCB Hair Products
(see Alberto-Culver Co.)

♥ TCCD Int'l, Inc. ■
3012 NW 25th Ave.
Pompano Beach, FL 33062
(800)653-4006, (954)960-4904
Personal care

♥ Tea Tree Icy Mineral Gel
(see Jason Natural Products)

▼ Teen Spirit
(see Colgate-Palmolive Co.)

▼ Tegrin® Shampoo
(see Block Drug Co.)

▼ Tek
(see Playtex Products, Inc.)

◆ Tender Touch
(see Aloette Cosmetics, Inc.)

♥ Ten-O-Six
(see Bonne Bell, Inc.)

♥ TerraNova®
(see AKA Saunders, Inc.)

♥ Terrapin Outdoor Systems, Inc. ■
P.O. Box 40339
Santa Barbara, CA 93140
(800)347-5211
Personal care

♥ TerrEssentials ■ ● ⊠
2650 Old National Pike
Middletown, MD 21769
(301)371-7333
Personal care, Household,
Companion animal

◆ Terry Binns SkinCare, Inc. ●
7301 Mission Rd., #106
Prairie Village, KS 66208
(800)909-7546, (913)722-6522
Personal care, Cosmetics

♥ Texas Best UnLimited, LP ✳ ■
P.O. Box 769
Kerrville, TX 78029-0769
(830)257-6020
Personal care

◆ Thera-Care Dip Additive
(see Espree Animal Products, Inc.)

▼ Thermasilk
(see Unilever United States Inc.)

◆ Third Millennium Science ✳ ■
7712 Rocio St.
Carlsbad, CA 92009
(800)776-6525, (760)431-7181
Personal care, Household,
Companion animal

▼ Tide
(see Procter & Gamble)

▼ Tilex
(see Clorox Company)

💗 Time Corrector® Firming
Moisture Cream
(see Jafra Cosmetics Int'l)

💗 Time Management Moisturizer
(see La Prairie, Inc.)

💗 Tisserand Aromatherapy
(see Avalon Natural Products)

▼ Toilet Duck Products
(see S.C. Johnson & Son, Inc.)

💗 Tomé Professional
Products, Inc. ✳ ■
P.O. Box 3388
Saratoga, CA 95070
(408)395-5425
Personal care

💗 tommy
(see Estee Lauder Companies)

💗 tommy girl
(see Estee Lauder Companies)

💗 Tommy Hilfiger Products
(see Estee Lauder Companies)

💗 Tom's of Maine, Inc. ■
P.O. Box 710
Kennebunk, ME 04043-0710
(800)367-8667, (207)985-2944
Personal care

💗 Tone®
(See Dial Corporation)

💗 Tools for Men
(see Change of Face Cosmetics)

▼ Top Guard
(see Marche Image Corp.)

▼ Top Job
(see Procter & Gamble)

💗 Topol Toothpaste
(see Schwarzkopf & Dep Inc.)

▼ Toujours Moi
(see Procter & Gamble)

❤ Tova Corp. ✳ ■
203 N. Aspan, Ste. 1
Azusa, CA 91702
(800)777-8682, (310)246-0218
Personal care, Cosmetics

❤ Trac II
(see Gillette Co.)

❤ Trend® Detergent
(see Dial Corporation)

▼ TRESemme Products
(see Alberto-Culver Co.)

◆ Tricia Bath and Body Shampoo
(see Aloette Cosmetics, Inc.)

❤ Triloka
(see Windrose Trading Co.)

❤ Tropez Cosmetics
(see AM Cosmetics, Inc.)

◆ Trophy Animal Health Care ✉
2796 Helen St.
Pensacola, FL 32504
(800)336-7087
Companion animal

◆ Tropical Botanicals ✳ ■
P.O. Box 635
Ramona, CA 92065
(760)788-4480
Personal care

▼ True Love
(see Elizabeth Arden Co.)

❤ Trutona and Harmonies
Feminine Products
(see BioProgress Technology, Ltd)

◆ TsP Powdered All Purpose Cleaner
(see America's Finest Products Corp.)

▼ Tuff Stuff
(see Clorox Company)

▼ Tuffy
(see Clorox Company)

❤ Tuscany
(see Estee Lauder Companies)

▼ Tussy
(see Playtex Products, Inc.)

❤ Two Star Dog ●
1370 10th St.
Berkeley, CA 94710
(510)525-1100
Personal care

▼ Two Thousand (2000)
Calorie Mascara
(see Procter & Gamble)

◆ U.S.A. Detergents ■ ●
1735 Jersey Ave.
North Brunswick, NJ 08902
(732)828-1800
Household

❤ Ultima II
(see Revlon, Inc.)

◆ Ultimate Bluing Shampoo
(see Espree Animal Products, Inc.)

◆ Ultimate Coat Conditioner
(see Espree Animal Products, Inc.)

❤ Ultimate Essential Mouth Care
(see Eco-Dent Int'l, Inc.)

▼ Ultra Brite
(see Colgate-Palmolive Co.)

❤ Ultra Glow Cosmetics ✳ ■ ● ⊠
P.O. Box 1469, Station A
Vancouver, BC, V6C 1P7
Canada
(604)444-4099
Personal care, Cosmetics

❦ Ultress
(see Clairol, Inc.)

❤ Uncommon Scents Inc. ■ ● ⊠
380 W. 1st Ave.
Eugene, OR 97401
(800)426-4336, (541)345-0952
Personal care

❤ Unelko Corp. ✳ ■
14641 N. 74th St.
Scottsdale, AZ 85260
(408)991-7272
Household

❤ Uni-Fresh® Air Freshener
(see Earth Friendly Products)

▼ Unilever United States Inc. ■
Lever House, 390 Park Ave.
New York, NY 10022
(800)598-1223, (212)888-1260
Personal care, Household

❤ Universal Light ✳ ■
P.O. Box 261
Wilmot, WI 53192-0261
(262)889-8571
Personal care

❤ un-petroleum Lip Care
(see Avalon Natural Products)

◆ Vademecum Toothpaste
(see Dermatone Lab Inc.)

◆ Vagosang Products
(see Ever Young, Inc.)

◆ Val-Chem Co. Inc. ✳ ■
P.O. Box 330
Sayre, PA 18840
(570)888-2285
Household

❤ Vanda Beauty Counselors, Inc. ▣
P.O. Box 3433
Orlando, FL 32802
(407)839-0223
Personal care, Cosmetics

▼ Vanish Bathroom Products
(see S.C. Johnson & Son, Inc.)

❤ Vano® Starch
(See Dial Corporation)

▼ Vaseline
(see Chesebrough-Pond's USA Co.)

🐾 Vavoom
(see Matrix Essentials, Inc.)

▼ Vel Soap
(see Colgate-Palmolive Co.)

▼ Venezia Fragrance
(see Procter & Gamble)

❤ Vermont Soapworks ■
616 Exchange St.
Middlebury, VT 05753
(802)388-4302
Personal care, Household

▼ Vibrance
(see Helene Curtis Int'l)

❤ Vicco Toothpaste
(see Universal Light)

❤ Victoria's Secret ■ ▣
P.O. Box 16586
Columbus, OH 43216
(614)856-6000
(see parent Limited, Inc.)
Personal care

▼ Vidal Sassoon ■
P.O. Box 599
Cincinnati, OH 45201
(513)983-1100
(see parent Procter & Gamble)
Personal care

♥ Vin-Dotco, Inc. ✳ ■
2875 MCI Dr.
Pinellas Park, FL 33782
(800)237-5911, (727)217-9200
Personal care, Household,
Companion animal

◆ Vita-Guard
(see Pro-Tec Pet Health)

☙ Vital Nutrients
(see Bristol-Myers Squibb Co.)

☙ Vitalis
(see Cairol, Inc)

◆ VitaWave ■
P.O. Box 5206
Ventura, CA 93005
(805)981-1472
Personal care

♥ VitaWave Colors and Perms
(see Beauty Naturally, Inc.)

▼ Vivid
(see Reckitt & Colman)

▼ VO5 Products
(see Alberto-Culver Co.)

♥ Voilé Parfumé
(see La Prairie, Inc.)

♥ Von Myering by Krystina ● ✉
208 Seville Ave.
Pittsburgh, PA 15214
(412)766-3186
Personal care

♥ V'tae Parfume & Body Care ■
576 Searls Ave.
Nevada City, CA 95959
(800)643-3011
Personal care

♥ Wachters' Organic Sea
Products Corp. ✳ ■
360 Shaw Rd.
South San Francisco, CA 94080
In CA (800)682-7100,
Outside CA (800)822-6565
Personal care, Household,
Companion animal

◆ Warm Earth Cosmetics ■ ▣
1155 Stanley Ave.
Chico, CA 95928-6944
(916)895-0455
Personal care, Cosmetics

▼ Warner-Lambert Co. ■
182 Tabor Rd.
Morris Plains, NJ 07950
(800)223-0182, (201)540-2000
Personal care

◆ Warren Laboratories, Inc. ■
12603 Executive Dr., Ste. 806
Stafford, TX 77477
(281)240-2563
Personal care, Cosmetics

◆ Wash 'N Curl
(see CCA Industries, Inc.)

▼ Wash n' Dri
(see Softsoap Enterprises)

❤ Waterman
(see Gillette Co.)

❤ Wave™ Dishwashing Liquid
(see Earth Friendly Products)

❤ Weleda, Inc. ■
175 N. Route, 9W
Congers, NY 10920
(914)268-8599
Personal care

❤ Wella Corporation ■
12 Mercedes Dr.
Montvale, NJ 07645
(201)930-1020
Personal care

❤ Wet 'N' Wild Cosmetics
(see AM Cosmetics, Inc.)

▼ Wet Ones
(see Playtex Products, Inc.)

◆ Whang Hall Products
(see Ever Young, Inc.)

◆ Whip-It Products, Inc. ✳ ■
P.O. Box 30128
Pensacola, FL 32503
(904)436-2125
Household

❤ White Linen
(see Estee Lauder Companies)

❤ White Rain
(see Gillette Co.)

❤ Whiteflower Analgesic Balm
(see Janta Int'l Co. (J.I.C.)

❤ Wild Bills Shaving Cream Bar Soap
(see Swan Lake Botanicals)

▼ Windex
(see S.C. Johnson & Son, Inc.)

❤ Windrose Trading Co. ✳ ●
P.O. Box 990
634 Schoolhouse Rd.
Madison, VA 22727
(540)948-2268
Household

▼ Windsong Fragrance
(see Chesebrough-Pond's USA Co.)

❤ Wings Fragrance
(see Giorgio Beverly Hills)

◆ Wipe Away Products
(see James Austin Co.)

❤ Wisdom Toothbrush Co. ●
2430 Payne St.
Evanston, IL 60201
(847)475-1439
Personal care

❤ WiseWays Herbals ■
Singing Brook Farm
99 Harvey Rd.
Worthington, MA 01098
(413)238-4268
Personal care, Household

▼ Wisk
(see Lever Brothers)

▼ Wizard Air Freshener
(see Reckitt & Colman)

❤ Womankind ✳ ■ ● ⌧
P.O. Box 1775
Sebastopol, CA 95473
(707)522-8662
Personal care

◆ Woodstock Natural
Products, Inc. ✳ ■
140 Sylvan Ave.
Englewood Cliff, NJ 07632
(800)615-6895
Personal care

▼ Woolite
(see Reckitt & Colman)

▼ Woolite Carpet and
Upholstery Cleaner
(see Playtex Products, Inc.)

❤ Wow-Bow Distributors, Ltd. ■ ● ⌧
13 B Lucon Dr.
Deer Park, NY 11729
(800)326-0230
Companion animal

❤ Wysong Corp. ■
1880 N. Eastman Rd.
Midland, MI 48640
(800)748-0188, (517)631-0009
Personal care, Companion animal

❤ XGel™ Products
(see BioProgress Technology, Ltd)

◆ Yardley of London ■
Building 9, Willow Lake Blvd.
Memphis, TN 38118
(901)547-7435
(see parent L'Oreal of Paris)
Personal care

▼ Yes
(see Reckitt & Colman)

❤ Yves Rocher, Inc. ■ ⊠
491 John Young Way, #300
Exton, PA 19341-2548
(800)321-YVES, (610)280-3200
Personal care, Cosmetics

❤ Zelda's ✳ ⊠
160 Esopus Ave.
Kingston, NY 12401
(800)647-8202
Personal care

❤ Zenith Is 4 The Planet ■ ● ⊠
P.O. Box 1739
Corvallis, OR 97339
(800)547-2741
Personal care, Household

▼ Zest
(see Procter & Gamble)

◆ Zhen, Inc. ● ⊠
P.O. Box 670
St. Francis, MN 55070
Cosmetics

❤ Zia Natural Skincare ■
1337 Evans Ave.
San Francisco, CA 94124
(800)334-7546, (415)642-8339
Personal care, Cosmetics

▼ Ziploc Products
(see S.C. Johnson & Son, Inc.)

◆ Zotos Int'l, Inc. ✳ ■ ⊠
100 Tokeneke Rd.
Darien, CT 06820-1005
(800)242-WAVE, (203)655-8911
Personal care, Cosmetics

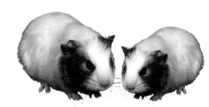

Parent Companies Behind Brand Names

The following list consists of **major** parent companies whose names may not be readily identifiable with their subsidiaries/divisions and brands. (For example, Tide is manufactured by Procter & Gamble.) This list is provided to help you become more familiar with the companies behind popular brand names, but is not inclusive of all companies and their subsidiaries and brands. Please keep in mind that companies, subsidiaries and divisions are continually being bought and sold and that individual subsidiaries and divisions within a company may have different testing policies. That's why it's best to refer to the main section of the book for specific information about a product or a brand name.

Key to Symbols Used

❤ Company is cruelty free. It DOES NOT test products or ingredients on animals, nor do any of its outside suppliers.

❥ Company DOES NOT test its products or ingredients on animals, but it is owned by a parent company that DOES test products and/or ingredients on animals.

◆ Company DOES NOT test its finished products or ingredients on animals, but has no agreement with its suppliers stating that they do not test their ingredients on animals.

▼ Company DOES test products or ingredients on animals.

DNR Company did not respond to *Personal Care* survey and therefore the testing status of this company is unknown. For a complete listing of companies that did not respond, see page 181.

▼ **3M**
Brands:
3M™, Dirtstop™ Mats, O-Cel-O™, Post-it® Notes, Scotch-Brite™, Scotchgard™, Scotch™ Magic™ Tape and Masking Tapes, Tarni-Shield™ Fine Metal Polishes, Trizact™ Abrasives

▼ Alberto-Culver Co.

Subsidiaries/Divisions:
St. Ives Laboratories(❦), Sally Beauty Company
Brands:
Alberto Styling Products, Bold Hold Products, Bone Strait, Consort Hair Products, Cortexx, FDS, Kleen Guard, Motions, Static Guard, Swiss Formula Hair & Skin Care Products, TCB Hair Products, TRESemme, TresGelee, TresHold, TresMend, TresPac, TresShine, TresWave II, VO5 Products

❤ Alexandra Avery Purely Natural Body Care

Brands:
Amberwoods Body Balsam, Dream Cream, Hawaiian Aloe Sun Oil, Jungle Blossoms Body Oil, Moonsilk Body Powder, Mountain Herbs Body Oil

◆ Amway

Brands:
Artistry® Skin Care & Cosmetics, Dish Drops® Concentrated Dishwashing Liquid, Glister®/Spreedent® Toothpaste, Glycerin & Honey Complexion Bar, L.O.C.® Multi-Purpose Cleaner, Moisture Essence Serum/Alpha Hydroxy Plus, SA8® Laundry Detergents

DNR Andrew Jergens Co.

Brands:
ActiBath® Treatments, Biore Facial Care Products, Curel, Jergens Naturals® with Aloe & Lanolin, Jergens Naturals® with Vitamin E & Chamomile, Jergens: Original Scent Lotion, Moisturizing Creamy Cleanser, Protective Moisture Lotion, Replenishing Moisture Lotion, Replenishing Vitamin E Lotion, Sensitive Skin Products, Shower Active® Moisturizer

▼ **Bausch & Lomb, Inc.**

Brands:

Boston® Brand, ReNu® Solution, Sensitive Eyes® Solution

DNR **Benckiser Consumer Products, Inc.**

Subsidiaries/Divisions:

Coty U.S. Inc.

Brands:

Aspen Cologne, Calgon Products, Cling Free Fabric Softener, Coty Products, Electrosol Detergent, Emeraude Perfume, Exclamation Perfume, Jet Dry Rinse Agent, Jovan Musk, Lime-A-Way, Preferred Stock Cologne, Stetson, Vanilla Fields, Vanilla Musk, Vanish

▼ **Block Drug Co.**

Brands:

Balmex® Diaper Rash Ointment, Polident® Denture Cleanser, Sensodyne® Toothpaste, Targon® Smokers' Mouthwash, Tegrin® Shampoo

❤ **Borlind of Germany**

Brands:

Annemarie Borlind, Baby Mild & Kind Care Cream, Blossom Dew Gel, Blossom Lotion, Body Lind, Ceramide Vital Fluid, Decollete Cream, For Lips, Herbal Facial Products, Intensive Care Capsules, Liposome Emulsion, Moisturizing Ampoule, Pura Soft, Pura Verde, Pure Radiance Candles, Ravenwood Essential Oils, Regeneration Ampoule, Regeneration Day Cream, Regeneration Night Cream, Seide Hair Care, Sportiv, SunLind, System Absolute, Touch-up Sticks, Ultra Gel, Ultra Stick, Velvet Creams

▼ Bristol-Myers Squibb Company

Subsidiaries/Divisions:
Clairol, Inc.(🐀), Matrix Essentials(🐀), Inc., Redmond Products, Inc.(🐀)
Brands:
12 Hour Hair Spray, 3 Minute Miracle, A Touch of Sun, Aussie All Over, Aussie Hair Do, Aussie Instant, Aussie Intermissions, Balsam Color, Barrier Reef, Beautiful Collection, Biolage, Blue Mountain Shampoo, Born Blonde, Citrifier, ColorMate, Curing Muddy, Daily Defense, DewPlex, Frizz Control, Frost & Tip, Hair Insurance, Hair Salad, Herbal Essences, Hydrience, Icon, Infusium 23, Instant Freeze Styling Spray, Keri, LacHydrin, Lasting Color by Loving Care, Logics, Loving Care, Mango Smoothy, Maxi Blonde Lightener, Maximum Hold Mousse, Mega Hair Products, Men's Choice, Miss Clairol, Moist, Moisturel, Natural Gel, Natural Instincts, Nice 'N Easy, Opticurl, Outback, Radiance, Rainforest, Real Volume Products, Revitalique, Sea Breeze, Skip-a-Step, Slip Detangler, Smoothy Products, Sprunch Spray, Ultress, Vavoom, Vital Nutrients, Vitalis

DNR Carter-Wallace, Inc.

Subsidiaries/Divisions:
Carter-Horner, Inc., Lambert-Kay
Brands:
Arrid Anti-perspirant Deodorant, First Response® pregnancy kit, Lady's Choice, Magnum Condoms, Nair® hair removal, Pearl Drops® tooth polish, Trojan® condoms

DNR Chattem, Inc.,

Brands:
Ban, Bull Frog Sunscreen, Corn Silk, Gold Bond, Mudd, Sun-In, Ultra Swim

▼ Church & Dwight Co., Inc.

Brands:

Arm & Hammer Baking Soda, Arm & Hammer Carpet & Room Deodorizer, Arm & Hammer Cat Litter Deodorizer, Arm & Hammer Super Scoop Clumping Cat Litter™, Arm & Hammer Deodorant, Brillo Pads, Bruce Floor Care, Cameo® Metal Polish, Dental Care® Products, Magic Sizing Starch, Parson's Ammonia, Parson's Bo-Peep Ammonia, Peroxicare® Toothpaste, Purex Toss N' Soft, Rain Drops, Sno Bol Drops, Sno Bowl Toilet Bowl Cleaner, Supreme Steel Wool

▼ Clorox Company

Subsidiaries/Divisions

A&M Products, Armor All Products Group, Brita (USA), First Brands, Kingsford Products Company, STP Corporation

Brands:

Armor All, Black Flag, Brita, Clorox 2, Clorox Products, Combat, EverClean, EverFresh, Formula 409, Fresh Step, Fresh Step Scoop, Glad, GladWare, Handi-Wipes, Heavy-Wipes, Jonny Cat, Kingsford, Lestoil, Liquid-Plumr, Match Light, No. 7, Pine-Sol, Rain Dance, Rally, S.O.S., Scoop Away, Soft Scrub, Stain Out, Tanner's Preserve, Tilex, Tilex Fresh Shower, Tuff Stuff, Tuffy

▼ Colgate-Palmolive

Subsidiaries/Divisions:

Hills' Pet Nutrition, Mennen Company, Murphy-Phoenix Co., Softsoap Enterprises

Brands:

Ajax, Baby Bath, Baby Magic, Balm Barr, Cashmere Bouquet, Colgate Instant Shave, Colgate Toothpastes, Curad, Dermassage, Dynamo, Fab, Fresh Start, Handi Wipes, Irish Spring, Javex Liquid Bleach, Kirkman Soap Products, Lady Speed Stick, Mersene Denture Cleaner, Murphy's Oil Soap, Palmolive, Prescription Diet, Protein 21 Shampoo & Hairspray, Protein 29 Hair Groom, Science Diet, Sesame St. Children's Bath Products, Skin Bracer, Softsoap Liquid Soap Products, Speed Stick, Teen Spirit, Ultra Brite, Vel Soap, Wash n' Dri

◆ Dr. A. C. Daniels

Brands:

Blue Lotion, Dermitite Lotion, Dog Ear Cleaner, Equinol Liquid Liniment, Gall Salve, Golden Shampoo, Heel Lotion, Hoof Ointment & Softener, Liquid Cat Wormer, Liquid Dog Wormer, Mitey Ear Cleaner, Skin Salve, Vapola Nasal Balm, Veterinary Petroleum Jelly, Wonder Lotion

◆ Del Laboratories, Inc.

Subsidiaries/Divisions:

Naturistics®, Quencher, Rejuvia, Sally Hansen

Brands:

Baby Orajel, Flame Glow Cosmetics, La Cross, N.Y.C. New York Color Cosmetics, Naturistics® Products, Orajel, Propha pH, Quencher Cosmetics, Rejuvia Vitamin E Skin Care Products, Sally Hansen Products

❤ Dial Corporation

Subsidiaries/Divisions:

Freeman Cosmetic Corp., Sarah Michael's, Inc.

Brands:

20 Mule Team® borax, Bare Foot, Borateem® bleach, Boraxo® soap, Breck® hair care products, Dial® Products, Dutch® detergent, Fels Naptha® soap, Freeman Hair & Skin Care Products, La France® brightener, Liquid Dial®, Nature's Accent®, Pure & Natural® soap, Purex Mountain Breeze® detergent, Purex®, Renuzit®, Sarah Michaels Bath & Body Products, StaFlo® starch, Tone®, Trend® detergent, Vano® starch

❤ Earth Friendly Products

Brands:

2 ply Bath Tissue, 2 ply Paper Towel, Cream Cleanser, Dishmate™, Earth Enzymes™, Ecos®, Fruit & Vegetable Wash, Furniture Polish, Non-Abrasive Orange Plus® Cleaning Towels, Orange Plus®, Orange Plus® Cleaning Towels, RTU Orange Plus®, Stain & Odor Remover, Toilet Bowl Cleaner, Uni Fresh Air Fresheners, Wave™, Window Kleener

❤ **Estee Lauder Companies, Inc.**

Subsidiaries/Divisions:

Aveda Corporation, MAC Cosmetics

Brands

Aramis, Aveda Products, Beautiful, Bobbi Brown Essentials, Clinique Beauty Products, Donna Karan Cosmetics, Freedom, Knowing, Lauder for Men, MAC Cosmetics, Origins Skin Care Products, Pleasures, Prescriptives Treatment & Cosmetic Products, Spellbound, tommy, tommy girl, Tommy Hilfiger Toiletries, Tuscany, White Linen

❤ **Frank T. Ross & Sons, Ltd.**

Brands:

Nature Clean Products (All Purpose Cleaning Lotion, Automatic Dishwasher Powder, Body Wash, Carpet & Upholstery Cleaner, Conditioner, Castille Hand Soap Liquid, Delicate Wash for Fine Fabrics, Fabric Softener, Kitchen & Bath Spray Cleaner, Floor Cleaner, Fruit & Veggie Wash, Laundry Stain Remover, Liquid Bleach Non Chlorine, Nature Clean Laundry Liquid, Non Chlorine Powdered Bleach, Non Toxic Oven Cleaner, Organic Laundry Powder, Shampoo, Soap Scum Remover, Toilet Bowl Cleaner, Tub & Tile Cream Cleanser, Wild Flower Window Glass Cleaner)

❤ **Gabriel Cosmetics, Inc.**

Brands:

Azulene Eye Make Up Remover, Banana Smoothie Detangler, Botanical Day & Night Moisturizer, Clean Kids Naturally (Shampoo, Detangler, Germ Busting Soap, Bubble Bath), Fango Sea Mud Mask, Gabriel Cosmetic Line, Oxygenating Cream, Invisible Gel, Tiny Bubbles Foaming Bath, Tropical Orange Burst Shampoo

❤ Gillette Company

Subsidiaries/Divisions:
Braun , Duracell, Inc., Oral-B Laboratories, Inc.

Brands:
Agility, Atra, Braun, CustomPlus, Daisy Shavers, Dippity-Do, Dry Idea, Duracell, Dynagrip, Eraser Mate, Face Saver, Foamy Shaving Cream, Gillette Shaving Series, Good News, Liquid Paper, MACH3 shaving system, Oral-B, Paper Mate, Parker, Right Guard, Satin Care Shaving Cream, SatinFloss, Sensor, SensorExcel for Women, Silkience, Soft & Dri, Tame, Trac II, Waterman, White Rain

▼ Johnson & Johnson

Subsidiaries/Divisions:
Neutrogena Corp.(❦), Personal Products Co.

Brands:
ACT Fluoride Rinse, Aveeno brand, Band-Aid, Carefree Panty Shields, Clean & Clear, Healthy Scalp®, Neutrogena Clean™, Neutrogena Products, o.b. tampons, On-The-Spot®, Purpose Moisturizer, Rainbath®, Reach Toothbrush, Shower to Shower, Stayfree, Sundown Sunscreen, Sure & Natural, T/Gel®, T/Scalp®

▼ Kimberly-Clark Corporation

Brands:
Cottonelle, Depend®, Hi-Dri Paper Towels, Huggies®, Kleenex®, Kotex®, Lightdays, New Freedom, Poise, Pull-Ups®, Scott Paper Co., Security Tampons

DNR Kiwi Brands, Inc.

Brands:
Ambi Skin Care, Behold Furniture Polish, Elite, Endust, Meltonian Shoe Care, Miracle White, Sneaker Shampoo, Sneaker White, Ty-D-Bol

◆ KMS Research

Brands:

AMP line, Color Vitality line, Curl Up line, Daily Repair line, Flat Out line, Hair Play line, Hair Stay line, Healthy Alternative line, Moisture Replace line, Puritives line, Silkier line

❤ L'anza Research Int'l

Brands:

Bodifying Cream, Body Styling Crème, Dramatic F/X, Finishing Freeze, Finishing Protector Dryspray, Fractals, Hardwire, L'anza, Mega Gel, Modify, Protecshine, Shine Gel, Software, Staitline, Styling Spritiz, Sure Success Acid Wave, Temporary Curl Relaxer and Smoother, Upgrade

◆ L'Oreal of Paris

Subsidiaries/Divisions:

Parfums Cacharel & Cie., Cosmair, Inc., Maybelline, Inc., Yardley of London, Laboratories Garnier, Lancome

Brands:

Biotherm Cosmetics & Skin Care, Cacharel Fragrances, Drakkar Noir, Georgio Armani Fragrances, Gloria Vanderbilt Fragrances, Guy Laroche Fragrances, Helena Rubenstein, L'Oreal Cosmetics, Lancome Cosmetics, Paloma Picasso Fragrances, Ralph Lauren Fragrances, Redken 5th Avenue, Yardley of London Skin Care Products

❤ Limited, Inc.

Subsidiaries/Divisions:

Bath & Body Works, Henri Bendel Inc., Victoria's Secret

Brands:

Bath & Body Works products, Rapture, Second Skin Satin

❤ Lotus Brands

Brands:

Alive Energy, Ancient Secrets, Ayate, Blue Pearl Incense, Color the Gray, Dragon Eggs, Harmony Pondicherry, Light Mountain Natural, Nature's Alchemy, Nirvana, Paul Penders Cosmetics, Rainforest Remedies, Sri Aurobindo Ashram, Sumeru Garden Herbals, Turtle Island Herbs

DNR LVMH Moet Hennessy Louis Vuitton

Subsidiaries/Divisions:

Guerlain, Inc., Christian Dior Perfumes, Inc., Parfums Givenchy, Inc.

Brands:

Dune Fragrance, Evolution Skincare, Fahrenheit Fragrance, Issima Skincare, Les Meteorites Cosmetics, L'Heure Bleue, Odelys Skincare, Poison Fragrance, Samsara Fragrance, Shalimar Fragrance, Terracotta Cosmetics

❤ Mar-Riche Enterprises, Inc.

Brands:

Bio Base, Coronation Anti-Wrinkle, Extra Riche, Fitness Shower Gel, Gerda Spillman Cosmetics & Skin Care, Hydro-Pearls, La Valeur De Spillman Fragrance, Mayfair Day Cream, Nail Elastic, Peau De Fleurs Cleansing Milk, Peau De Fleurs Facial Bar, Plantoseramin Lotion, Prestige Cream, R.A.O., Renaissance Bath Mousse, Rhythmic Massage Oil, Rosa Alpina, Skinmoist, Tagescreme, Tonique Sans Alcohol

❤ Mastey De Paris, Inc.

Brands:

Activateur Curl Enhancer, Activtan Tanning Accelerator, Affiné Cellulite Control, Basic Superpac Reconstructing Deep Conditioner, Clarté Creme Shampoo, Colour Refreshing Shampoo, Crémask Creme Facial Mask, Designer Liquid Mousse for Fine, Emulsioné Facial Cleanser, Enové Creme Shampoo, Enplacé Thickening Spray Gel For Fine, Eyecrém Anti-Wrinkle Crème, Fixé Finishing Spray for Fine, Fixé Super Hold Finishing Spray, Frehair Finishing Rinse, HC Formula + B5, Huiles

Essentielles Body Oil, L Hydraté Hand & Body Moiturizing Complex, L Stimulé Toning Mist, L'Exfoliant Facial Exfoliating Complex, Le Remouver Hair Clarifier, Liquid Pac, Lumineux Alcohol Free Shine Spray, Mastey Eau de Parfum, Mastey Men/Homme Eau de Cologne, Moisté Facial Moisturizer, Moisturée Moisturizing, Protége Hair Sunscreen, Regidé Maximum Hold Spritzer, Rejuvené Cellular Recovery Crème, Selftan Self-Tanning Crème, Shine Naturel Molding Lotion, SlimBody Slimming Complex, Sunbloc SPF 15 Sunscreen, Suncalm After Sun Relief, Suntan Creme SPF 4 Sunscreen, Swimmer's Shampoo, Swimmer's Shield, The Original LE GEL Products, Thin Hair Products, Traité Creme Shampoo, Velvetant Alpha Hydroxy Acid Skin Renewal Complex

◆ Neways Int'l
Brands:

1st Impression Cleanser, 2nd Chance Products, Barrier Cream, Bio-Mist Activator, Close Shaving Gel, Eliminator Mouthwash, Exhuberance Conditioner, Finishing Touch Hair Spray, Firm Up, Free Flex Hair Spray, Great Tan, Guardian Detergent/ Disinfectant, Gut Buster, Imperfect Lotion, Indulge Bubble Bath, Leslie DeeAnn Cosmetics, Leslie DeeAnn Nail Enamels, Lightning, Lipceutical, Milky Cleanser, NDK Gum, NewBrite Air Freshner & Deodorizer, NewBrite All Purpose Cleaner Concentrate, NewBrite Glass & Window Cleaner, NewBrite Hand Dish Soap Concentrate, NewBrite Liquid Laundry Detergent, Radiance Toothpaste, Rebound, Refresh Bath & Shower Gel, Refresh Bath/Shower Gel, Replenishing Mist, Retention Plus, Sassy Spritz/Spray Gel, Sculpting Gel, Silken Mild Family Shampoo, Snap Back, Sparkle Bathroom & Tile Cleaner, Subdue Deodorant, Sunbrero, Super S Cream, Super Booster, Super Skinny Dip, Tanacity, Tangible Massage Lotion, Tender Care Body Lotion, TLC Cleansing Lotion, Ultimate Shampoo, Whiten Tooth Whitener, Wrinkle Drops, Wrinkle Garde

❤ **Para Laboratories, Inc.**

Brands:

Alogoli Soap, Argile Blanche Soap, Argile Rose Soap, Argilet Soap, Argimiel Soap, Cholesterol Hair Care Products, Crystalene Clear Gel, Garlic Hair Care Products, Gift of Life Creme, Hair & Scalp Dressing, Le Stick Deodorant, Mint Julip Products, Mud Pack Masque, Old Western Hair & Scalp Treatment, Perm-Last Spray-In Conditioner, Placenta Hair Care Products, Pro-Rich Conditioning Gel, Queen Helene Products, Rum 'N Egg Shampoo, RX-18 Shampoo, Soft 'N Shine, Super Cholesterol Hair Conditioner, Super Protein 4 in 1 Conditioner & Sty Gel

◆ **Parlux Fragrances, Inc.**

Brands:

Animale for Women, Animale for Men, Animale Animale for Women, Animale Animale for Men, Instinct d'Animale for Women, Baryshnikov for Women, Baryshnikov for Men, Baryshnikov Sport, Hollywood for Women, Hollywood for Men, Fred Hayman's Touch for Women, Fred Hayman's Touch for Men, 273 for Women, 273 for Men, Portfolio, Reserve, America for Women, America for Men, 360 for Women, 360 for Men, Perry Ellis for Women, Perry Ellis for Man

◆ **Patricia Allison**

Brands:

Babyskin Masque, Beauty Banquet Lecitmol, French Strawberry Creme Cleanser, Irism Legend Hand Creme, Nutrient Balm, Oasis Moisture Balm, Peppermint Pickup Stimulation Masque, Petalskin Hand & Body Balm, Roman Oil Beauty Bath, Rose Petal Luxury Shampoo & Body Wash, Shimmer Hair Conditioner, Swedish Scrub, Un-Line, Vita Balm, Vita Magic Night Creme, Wild Fern Freshener

▼ **Playtex Products**

Brands:

Banana Boat, Better Off, Binanca, BioSun, Chubs, Dentax, Diaparene, Dorothy Gray, Jhirmack Hair Care Products, La Coupe, Mr. Bubble, Ogilvie, Playtex® Tampons, Tek, Tussy, Wet Ones, Woolite Carpet and Upholstery Cleaner

▼ **Procter & Gamble Co.**

Subsidiaries/Divisions:

Clarion Cosmetics, Cover Girl Cosmetics, Giorgio Beverly Hills, Max Factor, Noxell Corp., Olay Co., Inc., The Pantene Co., Procter & Gamble Cosmetics Co., Tambrands, Inc., Vidal Sassoon, Richardson-Vicks, Inc.

Brands:

Always, Attends, Bain de Soleil, Banner, Biz, Bold, Bounce, Bounty, Camay, Cascade, Charmin, Cheer, Clarion Cosmetics, Clearasil, Coast, Comet, Cover Girl Cosmetics, Crest, Dash Detergent, Dawn, Downy, Dreft, Dryel Fabric Care, Era, Febreze Fabric Spray, Gain, Giorgio Beverly Hills Products, Gleem Toothpaste, Head & Shoulders, Hugo Boss Fragrance, Incognito, Ivory, Joy, Kleenite, Laura Biagiotti-Roma, Lava, Luvs, Max Factor Cosmetics, Mr. Clean, Navy, Noxema, Oil of Olay, Old Spice, Oxydol, Pampers, Pantene, Pert Plus, Prell, Puffs, Red Fragrance, Safeguard, Scope, Secret, Spic & Span, Sure, Swiffer Sweeper, Tampax Tampons, Tide, Top Job, Venezia Fragrance, Vidal Sassoon Products, Wings Fragrance, Zest

▼ **Reckitt & Colman Inc.**

Brands:

Chore Boy, d-Con, Dettol, Easy-Off, Glass Plus, Lysol, Mop & Glo, Neet, Old English, Resolve, Sani-Flush, Snowy, Spray 'n Wash, Stick-Ups, Vivid, Wizard Air Freshener, Woolite, Yes

❤ Revlon, Inc.

Subsidiaries/Divisions:

Almay, Inc., Bill Blass, Inc., Carrington Parfums Ltd., Charles of the Ritz Group Ltd., The Cosmetic Center Inc., Halston Enterprises, Inc., Lancaster Inc., Norell Perfumes, Inc., Prestige Perfumes Ltd., The Princess Marcella Borghese, Inc.

Brands:

African Pride, Age Defying Makeup, Almay, Bill Blass Products, Borghese Cosmetics, Carrington Parfums, Charles of the Ritz Products, Charlie, ColorStay®, Fire & Ice, Flex, Germaine Monteil Cosmetics, Halston Products, Jean Nate, Jeanne Gatineau Fragrance, Jontue, Lady Mitchum, Lancaster Products, Mitchum, No Sweat, Norell Fragrances, Outrageous™, Princess Marcella Borghese Products, Streetwear, Ultima II

▼ S.C. Johnson & Son, Inc.

Brands:

Armstrong Floor Cleaner, Brite, Deep Woods OFF!, Drano Products, Edge Shaving Products, Fantastik, Favor, Fine Wood One-Step, Fine Wood Paste Wax, Future, Glade Products, Glo-Coat, Glory, Jubilee Spray, Klean 'n Shine, OFF!, OFF! Skintastic, Pledge, Raid Products, Rhuli Products, Saran Wrap, Scrubbing Bubbles, Shout Carpet Cleaner, Shout Soil & Stain Remover, Shower Shine, Skintimate Shaving Products, Step Saver, Toilet Duck Products, Vanish Products, Windex, Ziploc Products

❤ Scruples Professional Salon Products, Inc.

Brands:

Cohesion Intercellular Hair Binder, Effects Hair Products, Emphasis Texturing Styling Mousse, Enforce Hair Products, ER Emergency Repair for Damaged Hair, In Protein Spray, Moisture Bath Shampoo, Moisturex Intensive Moisture Treatment, More Emphasis Styling Mousse, O2 Hair Products, Quickseal Fortifying Creme Conditioner, REconstruct Leave, Renewal Hair Products, Smooth Out Hair Products, Snafu Styling Stick, Spray Lites Hair Glosser, Structure Bath Shampoo, Tea Tree Sculpting Gel, Total Accents Precision Creme, Ultra Form Molding Spray, V2 Double Volume for Hair

❤ Seventh Generation
Brands:

All Purpose Cleaner, Bathroom Tissues, Full Spectrum Light Bulbs, Glass Cleaner, Non-Chlorine Bleach, Paper Plates, Paper Towels, Plastic Trash Bags, Toilet Bowl Cleaner, Ultra Fabric Softener, Ultra Laundry Liquid, Ultra Laundry Powder

▼ SmithKline Beecham Consumer Healthcare
Brands:

Aquafresh Toothpaste, Dr. Best, Glysolid Cream, Massengill Products

❤ Tom's of Maine, Inc.
Brands:

Natural Baby Shampoo, Natural Toothpaste for Children, Natural Toothpaste for Sensitive Teeth, Natural Flossing Ribbon, Natural Mouthwash, Natural Baking Soda Mouthwash, Natural Deodorant, Natural Antiperspirant Deodorant, Natural Shampoo with Aloe & Almond, Natural Shaving Cream, Natural Deodorant Soap, Natural Moisturizing Soap, Natural Glycerin Soap

▼ Unilever United States, Inc.
Subsidiaries/Divisions:

Calvin Klein Cosmetics Co., Chesebrough-Pond's USA Co., Elizabeth Arden Co., Helene Curtis International, Lever Brothers Co., Parfums International Ltd.

Brands:

5th Avenue, Aim, All, Aqua Net, Aviance, Aviance Night Musk, Aziza, Babe, Blue Grass, Breeze, Brut Products, Cachet, Caress, Chloe, cK be, cK one, Close-Up, Contradiction, Cutex, Degree, Disney Toothbrushes, Dove, Elizabeth Taylor White Diamonds, Escape, Eternity, Faberge, Final Touch Dryer Sheets, Finesse, Impulse, Lagerfeld, Lagerfeld Jako, Lever 2000, Lifebuoy, Lux, Mentadent, Obsession, Passion, Pepsodent, Ponds, Power Stick, Prince Matchabelli, Q-Tips Products, Quantum, Rave, Red Door, Rinso, Salon Selectives, Shield, Signal Mouthwash, Snuggle, Splendor, Suave, Sunflowers, Sunlight, Surf, Thermasilk, True Love, Vaseline, Very Valentino, Vibrance, White Diamond, White Shoulders, Windsong, Wisk

▼ Warner-Lambert Company

Subsidiaries/Divisions:
Parke-Davis Company
Brands:
Corn Huskers Lotion, E.P.T. Early Pregnancy Test, Efferdent, Fresh 'n Brite, Listerine, Listermint, Lubriderm, Schick, Three Flowers

❤ WiseWays Herbals

Brands:
All Heal Salve, Arabian Amber, Beautiful Belly Balm, Bug Ease, Detox Bath Crystals, Enchanted Forest, Fabulous Fennel Face Balm & Scrub, Grandmother Moon Balm, Jade Forest After Shave, Lavender Burn Spray, Mists of Pleasure Laundry Freshener, Mother's Happy Child, Raven & Golden Apple Cider Vinegar Rinses, Rites of Romance, Sava Foot Soak, Selena Massage Oil, Sparkle My Spirit, Sweet Annie Vinegar Douche, Sweet Cicely Furniture Polish, Tea Tree Foot Powder

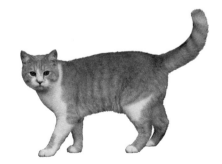

❤ Guide to Cruelty-Free ❤
Products by Product Type

This section will assist you in finding specific types of products manufactured by cruelty-free companies listed in this book. Due to space constraints, products are listed by the name of the companies that manufacture them, not by individual brand names. To find out who manufactures or distributes a particular brand name product, check the listings in the front of the book.

AIR FRESHENERS

Amazon Premium
    Products
American Eco-Systems
Anthe-Essence
    Aromatherapy
Aphrodisia Products
Auroma Int'l
Bath Island
Celestial Body
Clear Light The Cedar Co.
Dial Corporation
Earth Friendly Products
Earthly Matters
Garden Botanika
Herb Garden
Herbal Products &
    Development
Hummers
Indigo Wild Aromatics
Lotus Brands
McAuley's

Mia Rose Products
Native Scents
Neo Tech Cosmetic
Prima Fleur Botanicals
Sarah Michaels
Shadow Lake
Vermont Soapworks
WiseWays Herbals
Wysong Corp.

AROMATHERAPY

Abra Therapeutics
Ahimsa Natural Beauty
Alexandra Avery Purely
    Natural Body Care
Amrita Aromatherapy
Anthe-Essence
    Aromatherapy
Aphrodisia Products
Appleberry Attic
Arbico Environmentals
Arizona Natural Resources

Aroma Life
Aroma Terra
Aroma Vera
Aromaland
Auroma Int'l
Avalon Natural
    Products
Avon Products
Bare Escentuals
Bath & Body Works
Bath Island
Bavarian Alpenol &
    Sunspirit
Belle Star
Body & Soul
    Aromatherapy
Body Crystal Environ-
    mental Products
Body Shop
Burt's Bees
C.E. Hinds
CA-Botana Int'l

California Baby Botanical Skin Care
CD&P Health Products
Celestial Body
Chishti
Clientele
Colin Ingram
Colour Energy Corp.
Deodorant Stones of America (D.S.A.)
Derma E
Earth Science
East End Imports
Elizabeth Van Buren Aromatherapy
Exotic Nature Body Care Products
Faith Products
Flower Essence Services
Gabriel Cosmetics
Herb Garden
Heritage Store
Honeybee Gardens
Hummers
Indigo Wild Aromatics
Innovative Body Science
Izy's Aromatherapy Skin Care & Holistic Cosmetics
Jason Natural Products
Kettle Care
Khepra Skin Care
Kim Manley Herbals

La Dove
Lady of the Lake
Lakon Herbals
Lily of Colorado
Limited
Lotus Brands
Lunar Farms Herbal Specialist
Magic of Aloe
Maharishi Ayur-Veda Products
Master's Flower Essences
McAuley's
Mera Personal Care Products
Mia Rose Products
Mountain Rose Herbs
Nadina's Cremes
Native Scents
Natural Bodycare
NaturElle Cosmetics
Nature's Apothacary
Nature's Sunshine Products
North Country Glycerine Soap
Philip B. Hair & Body Care
Precious Collection Aromatherapy
Prima Fleur Botanicals
Pure Touch Therapeutics
Ravenwood

Secret Gardens
Shadow Lake
Siddha Int'l
Simpler Thyme®
Simplers Botanical
Smith & Vandiver
St. John's Herb Garden
Starwest Botanicals
Sumeru Garden Herbals
Sunfeather Natural Soap
Surrey
Swan Lake Botanicals
TerrEssentials
Tova Corp.
Uncommon Scents
Vermont Soapworks
V'tae Parfume & Body Care
Wachters' Organic Sea Products Corp.
WiseWays Herbals
Wow-Bow Distributors
Yves Rocher

BABY PRODUCTS

ADWE Laboratories
Ahimsa Natural Beauty
Aloe Creme Laboratories
Arbico Environmentals
Aroma Terra
Aroma Vera
Aubrey Organics
Bath Island

Body Crystal Environmental Products
Borlind of Germany
Burt's Bees
California Baby Botanical Skin Care
Dreamous Corp.
Earth Science
Faith Products
Flower Essence Services
Gabriel Cosmetics
Great Mother's Goods
H2O Plus
Heritage Store
Indigo Wild Aromatics
Innovative Body Science
Kettle Care
Kiehl's
Kim Manley Herbals
La Dove
Lakon Herbals
Levlad /Nature's Gate
Little Forest Natural Baby Products
Logona USA
Lotus Brands
Lunar Farms Herbal Specialist
Maharishi Ayur-Veda Products
Montagne Jeunesse
Motherlove herbal
Mountain Rose Herbs

Nadina's Cremes
North Country Glycerine Soap
Prima Fleur Botanicals
Real Aloe
Reviva Labs
Shaklee Corp.
Simmons Natural Bodycare
Smith & Vandiver
Sumeru Garden Herbals
Sunfeather Natural Soap
TerrEssentials
Tom's of Maine
Vermont Soapworks
Weleda
WiseWays Herbals

BATH PRODUCTS
Abra Therapeutics
ADWE Laboratories
Ahimsa Natural Beauty
Alaska Herb & Tea
Allens Naturally
Aloe Creme Laboratories
Alvin Last
Amazon Premium Products
American Eco-Systems
American Formulating & Mfg.
Anthe-Essence Aromatherapy

Aphrodisia Products
Appleberry Attic
Arbico Environmentals
Arizona Natural Resources
Aroma Terra
Aroma Vera
Aromaland
Aubrey Organics
Auroma Int'l
Avalon Natural Products
Bare Escentuals
Bath & Body Works
Bath Island
Beehive Botanicals
Belle Star
Bio Pac
Biogime Int'l
Bi-O-Kleen Industries
BioProgress Technology
Body & Soul Aromatherapy
Body Crystal Environmental Products
Body Shop
Bodyography
Borlind of Germany
CA-Botana Int'l
California Baby Botanical Skin Care
California Mango
Canada's All Natural Soap
CD&P Health Products
Celestial Body

Chishti
Clarins of Paris
Classic Cosmetics
Clearly Natural Products
Clientele
Colora Henna
Colour Energy Corp.
Dial Corporation
Dr. Bronner's
  Magic Soaps
Earth Friendly Products
Earth Science
Earthly Matters
Elizabeth Van Buren
  Aromatherapy
Espial USA
Exotic Nature Body
  Care Products
Faith Products
Flower Essence Services
Flowery Beauty Products
Freeman Cosmetic Corp.
French Transit
Gabriel Cosmetics
Gap
Garden Botanika
Gillette
Great Mother's Goods
H2O Plus
Helen Lee Skin Care
  & Cosmetics
Herb Garden
Heritage Store

Hewitt Soap
Honeybee Gardens
Hummers
Indigo Wild Aromatics
Innovative Body Science
J & J Jojoba/California
  Gold Products
Jackie Brown Cosmetics
Jamieson Laboratories
Jelmar
JOICO Labs
Kettle Care
Kim Manley Herbals
KSA Jojoba
La Dove
Lady of the Lake
Lakon Herbals
Lan-O-Sheen
Levlad/Nature's Gate
Limited
Little Forest Natural
  Baby Products
Logona USA
Lotus Brands
Lunar Farms Herbal
  Specialist
Magic of Aloe
Marilyn Miglin L.P.
Mar-Riche Enterprises
Master's Flower Essences
McAuley's
Meta Int'l
Montagne Jeunesse

Mountain Rose Herbs
Murad
NAACO
Nadina's Cremes
Native Scents
Natural Bodycare
Neo Tech Cosmetic
Nirvana
Norimoor
North Country
  Glycerine Soap
Ohio Hempery
Para Laboratories
Penny Island Products
Person & Covey
Pharmagel Corp.
Prima Fleur Botanicals
Pure Touch Therapeutics
Rainbow Research
Ravenwood
Real Aloe
Redmond Minerals
Revlon
Roebic Laboratories
Safe Solutions
Sappo Hill Soapworks
Sarah Michaels
Schwarzkopf & Dep
Seventh Generation
Shadow Lake
Shaklee Corp.
ShiKai Products
Sierra Dawn Products

Simmons Natural
    Bodycare
Simpler Thyme®
Smith & Vandiver
Soap Factory
St. John's Herb Garden
Starwest Botanicals
Sterling Clean
Sumeru Garden Herbals
Surrey
Swan Lake Botanicals
TerrEssentials
Tom's of Maine
Tova Corp.
Uncommon Scents
Unelko Corp.
Vermont Soapworks
Victoria's Secret
Wachters' Organic
    Sea Products Corp.
Weleda
WiseWays Herbals
Wysong Corp.
Yves Rocher
Zenith Is 4 The Planet

BATHROOM CLEANERS
ADWE Laboratories
Allens Naturally
Amazon Premium Products
American Eco-Systems
Arbico Environmentals
Aubrey Organics

Bath Island
Bio Pac
Bi-O-Kleen Industries
Body Crystal Environ-
    mental Products
Dial Corporation
Dr. Bronner's Magic Soaps
Earth Friendly Products
Earthly Matters
Espial USA
Faith Products
Hummers
Jelmar
McAuley's
NAACO
Natural Bodycare
Roebic Laboratories
Shadow Lake
Shaklee Corp.
Sierra Dawn Products
Simmons Natural
    Bodycare
Soap Factory
Sterling Clean
Unelko Corp.
Vermont Soapworks
Zenith Is 4 The Planet

CARPET/RUG CARE
Amazon Premium Products
American Formulating
    & Mfg.
Arbico Environmentals

Bi-O-Kleen Industries
Dial Corporation
Earthly Matters
Espial USA
Frank T. Ross & Sons
Hummers
Kyjen
Lan-O-Sheen
McAuley's
NAACO
Shadow Lake
Soap Factory

COMPANION
ANIMAL CARE
Allerpet
Amazon Premium Products
Appleberry Attic
Arbico Environmentals
Aubrey Organics
Ayurveda Holistic Center
Bath Island
Baxter Environmental
    Products DBA Nala
    Berry Laboratories
Bi-O-Kleen Industries
Body Crystal Environ-
    mental Products
Brookside Soap
Burt's Bees
Canada's All Natural
    Soap
Danklied Laboratories

Dr. Goodpet
Eqyss Int'l
Fleabusters/Rx for Fleas
Flower Essence Services
Green Ban
Herb Garden
Hummers
Indigo Wild Aromatics
KSA Jojoba
Kyjen
Mallory Pet Supplies
Master's Flower Essences
MediPatch Laboratories
Mountain Rose Herbs
Nadina's Cremes
North Country
   Glycerine Soap
PetGuard
Redmond Minerals
Safe Solutions
Simmons Natural Bodycare
Soap Works
Sojourner Farms
Solid Gold Health
   Products for Pets
St. JON Laboratories
Sunfeather Natural Soap
Swan Lake Botanicals
TerrEssentials
Vermont Soapworks
Vin-Dotco
Wachters' Organic Sea
   Products Corp.

Wow-Bow Distributors
Wysong Corp.

CONDOMS
Nadina's Cremes

CONTACT
LENS CARE
Clear Conscience LLC
Prima Fleur Botanicals

COSMETICS
Absolute Aloe Int'l.
ADWE Laboratories
Almay, Inc.
Aloe Complete
Aloe Creme
   Laboratories
AM Cosmetics
Amazon Premium
   Products
American Int'l Ind.
Amrita Aromatherapy
Arbico Environmentals
Arizona Natural Resources
Aroma Life
Aubrey Organics
Auroma Int'l
Avalon Natural Products
Aveda Corporation
Avon Products
Bare Escentuals
Bath & Body Works

Benetton USA Corp.
Bob Kelly Cosmetics
Body Crystal Environ-
   mental Products
Body Shop
Bodyography
Bonne Bell
Borlind of Germany
C.E. Hinds
Catherine Atzen
   Laboratories
Chanel
Clarins of Paris
Classic Cosmetics
Clear Light The Cedar Co.
Clientele
Colora Henna
D.K. USA
Dena Corp.
Deodorant Stones of
   America (D.S.A.)
Derma-Life Corp.
Discount Deodorant
   Stones
Dreamous Corp.
Earth Science
Espial USA
Estee Lauder Companies
Flowery Beauty Products
Freeman Cosmetics Corp.
Gabriel Cosmetics
Gap
Garden Botanika

Gena Laboratories
Gillette
Giovanni Hair
    Care Products
H2O Plus
Health and Body Fitness
Helen Lee Skin Care
    & Cosmetics
Henry Bendel, Inc.
Heritage Store
Island Dog
Izy's Aromatherapy
    Skin Care & Holistic
    Cosmetics
J & J Jojoba/California
    Gold Products
J. Stephen Scherer
Jacki's Magic Lotion
Jackie Brown Cosmetics
Jafra Cosmetics Int'l
Jamieson Laboratories
Jelene
Kiehl's
Kiss My Face Corp.
KSA Jojoba
La Crista
La Prairie
Lily of Colorado
Limited
Logona USA
Lotus Brands
MAC Cosmetics
Mad Gab's

Magic of Aloe
Margarite Cosmetics/
    Moon Products
Marilyn Miglin L.P.
Mar-Riche Enterprises
Mary Kay Cosmetics
Mastey De Paris
Merle Norman
    Cosmetics
Meta Int'l
Montagne Jeunesse
Mountain Ocean
Mountain Rose Herbs
Murad
Nadina's Cremes
NaturElle Cosmetics
Norimoor
Nutri-Cell
OPI Products
Orlane
Orly International
Pharmagel Corp.
Prima Fleur Botanicals
Real Natural Products
Reviva Labs
Revlon
Rexall Showcase Int'l
Sea Minerals
Shaklee Corp.
Siddha Int'l
Sombra Cosmetics
Swan Lake Botanicals

TaUT by Leonard
    Engelman
Tova Corp.
Ultra Glow Cosmetics
Yves Rocher
Zia Natural Skincare

DENTAL CARE
ADWE Laboratories
Aloe Creme Laboratories
Alvin Last
Arbico Environmentals
Auroma Int'l
Bath Island
Beehive Botanicals
Body Crystal Environ-
    mental Products
Body Tools
Dreamous Corp.
Eco-Dent Int'l
Espial USA
Gillette
Heritage Store
Hummers
Levlad/Nature's Gate
Logona USA
Lotus Brands
Maharishi Ayur-
    Veda Products
Mountain Rose Herbs
Nature's Sunshine Products
Norimoor
Peelu

Penn Herb
Prima Fleur Botanicals
Schwarzkopf & Dep
Shaklee Corp.
Tom's of Maine
Universal Light
Weleda
Wysong Corp.

DEODORANTS/ ANTIPERSPIRANTS
Abkit
Alvin Last
Arbico Environmentals
Aroma Life
Aubrey Organics
Avalon Natural Products
Avon Products
Bath Island
Body Crystal Environmental Products
Borlind of Germany
Celestial Body
Clarins of Paris
Deodorant Stones of America (D.S.A.)
Discount Deodorant Stones
Earth Science
Espial USA
Faith Products
French Transit
Gap

Gillette
H2O Plus
Heritage Store
Honeybee Gardens
Hummers
Innovative Body Science
Izy's Aromatherapy Skin Care & Holistic Cosmetics
Jason Natural Products
Kettle Care
Levlad/Nature's Gate
Logona USA
Mar-Riche Enterprises
Neo Tech Cosmetic
Para Laboratories
Penn Herb
Revlon
Shaklee Corp.
Sumeru Garden Herbals
TCCD Int'l
TerrEssentials
Texas Best UnLimited
Tom's of Maine
Weleda
WiseWays Herbals
Wysong Corp.
Yves Rocher

FEMININE HYGIENE
Arbico Environmentals
BioProgress Technology
Earth Science

Hummers
Les Femmes
Lotus Pads
Mountain Rose Herbs
Natracare
Organic Essentials
Simmons Natural Bodycare
Womankind

FIRST AID
Arbico Environmentals
Aubrey Organics
Beehive Botanicals
Carma Laboratories
Danklied Laboratories
Derma E
Derma-Life Corp.
Earth Science
Espial USA
Flower Essence Services
Heritage Store
Hobe Laboratories
Jamieson Laboratories
Kim Manley Herbals
Lotus Brands
Mountain Rose Herbs
WiseWays Herbals

FOOT CARE
Abra Therapeutics
Aloe Creme Labs
Alvin Last

Amazon Premium Products
American Int'l Ind.
American Safety Razor
Aphrodisia Products
Arbico Environmentals
Aubrey Organics
Bare Escentuals
Bavarian Alpenol & Sunspirit
Body & Soul Aromatherapy
Bodyography
Burt's Bees
CA-Botana Int'l
Deodorant Stones of America (D.S.A.)
Derma E
Dial Corporation
Earth Science
Espial USA
Faith Products
Flowery Beauty Products
Freeman Cosmetic Corp.
Garden Botanika
Gena Laboratories
Heritage Store
Hummers
Innovative Body Science
Jamieson Laboratories
Kettle Care
Khepra Skin Care
Kim Manley Herbals

KSA Jojoba
La Dove
Lotus Brands
Mar-Riche Enterprises
Montagne Jeunesse
Mountain Rose Herbs
Natural Bodycare
NaturElle Cosmetics
Norimoor
Para Laboratories
Prima Fleur Botanicals
Remington Products
Reviva Labs
Shaklee Corp.
Simmons Natural Bodycare
Smith & Vandiver
Soap Factory
Starwest Botanicals
TCCD Int'l
TerrEssentials
Tova Corp.
Vermont Soapworks
Weleda
WiseWays Herbals
Yves Rocher

FRAGRANCES

Amazon Premium Products
American Int'l Ind.
Amrita Aromatherapy
Aphrodisia Products

Appleberry Attic
Arbico Environmentals
Aroma Terra
Aromaland
Aubrey Organics
Auroma Int'l
Avon Products
Bare Escentuals
Bath & Body Works
Bath Island
Belle Star
Benetton USA Corp.
Body Crystal Environmental Products
Body Shop
Bonne Bell
Burt's Bees
Chanel
Chishti
Clarins of Paris
Clear Light The Cedar Co.
D.K. USA
Deodorant Stones of America (D.S.A.)
Earth Science
East End Imports
Estee Lauder
Exotic Nature Body Care Products
Flower Essence Services
Gap
Garden Botanika
Gillette

Great Mother's Goods
H2O Plus
Henri Bendel
Herb Garden
Heritage Store
Honeybee Gardens
Hummers
Indigo Wild Aromatics
Innovative Body Science
Kettle Care
Kiehl's
KSA Jojoba
La Prairie
Limited
Lotus Brands
Marilyn Miglin L.P.
Mar-Riche Enterprises
Mary Kay Cosmetics
Mastey De Paris
McAuley's
Mia Rose Products
Mountain Rose Herbs
Nadina's Cremes
Prima Fleur Botanicals
Pure Touch Therapeutics
Ravenwood
Revlon
Secret Gardens
Shaklee Corp.
Siddha Int'l

Simmons Natural Bodycare
Smith & Vandiver
Soap Factory
St. John's Herb Garden
Starwest Botanicals
Sumeru Garden Herbals
Tova Corp.
Uncommon Scents
V'tae Parfume & Body Care
Victoria's Secret
WiseWays Herbals
Yves Rocher

FURNITURE POLISHES/WAXES/CLEANERS

Amazon Premium Products
Earth Friendly Products
Frank T. Ross & Sons
Hummers
JC Garet
Jelmar
McAuley's
NAACO
Seventh Generation
Simmons Natural Bodycare
WiseWays Herbals
Zenith Is 4 The Planet

HAIR CARE

ABBA Pure & Natural Hair Care
Abkit
Advanced Research Labs
ADWE Laboratories
Ahimsa Natural Beauty
Alexandra Avery Purely Natural Body Care
Allon Personal Care
Aloe Commodities
Alvin Last
American Int'l Ind.
Appleberry Attic
Arbico Environmentals
Aroma Terra
Aroma Vera
Aubrey Organics
Avalon Natural Products
Avon Products
Bare Escentuals
Bath & Body Works
Bath Island
Beauty Naturally
Beehive Botanicals
Bio Pac
Body & Soul Aromatherapy
Body Shop
Bonne Bell
Borlind of Germany
Burt's Bees
CA-Botana Int'l
Catherine Atzen Laboratories

Celestial Body
Chuckles
Clairol
Clarins of Paris
Clear Light The
    Cedar Co.
Clientele
Colora Henna
Dena Corp.
Derma-Life Corp.
Earth Science
Espial USA
Faith Products
Framesi USA/Roffler
Frank T. Ross & Sons
Freeman Cosmetic Corp.
Gabriel Cosmetics
Gap
Garden Botanika
Gillette
Giovanni Hair Care
    Products
H2O Plus
Health and Body
    Fitness
Helen Lee Skin Care
    & Cosmetics
Herb Garden
Heritage Store
Hobe Laboratories
Honeybee Gardens
Hummers
Innovative Body Science

Institute of Trichology
J & J Jojoba/California
    Gold Products
Jason Natural Products
Jelene
John Amico Expressive
    Hair Care Products
John Frieda Professional
    Hair Care
John Paul
    Mitchell Systems
JOICO Labs
Kiehl's
Kim Manley Herbals
Kiss My Face Corp.
La Dove
Lan-O-Sheen
Logona USA
Lotus Brands
Magic of Aloe
Mary Kay Cosmetics
Matrix Essentials
McAuley's
Mera Personal Care Products
Montagne Jeunesse
Mountain Ocean
Mountain Rose Herbs
Natural Bodycare
Natural Nectar Corp.
NaturElle Cosmetics Corp.
Nature's Sunshine Products
Neo Tech Cosmetic
Nexxus Products

Nirvana
North Country
    Glycerine Soap
Nutraceutical Corp.
Ohio Hempery
Para Laboratories
Penny Island Products
Person & Covey
Pharmagel Corp.
Prima Fleur Botanicals
Rainbow Research Corp.
Rainforest
Real Aloe
Redmond Products
Remington Products
Reviva Labs
Revlon
Safe Solutions
Schwarzkopf & Dep
Scruples Professional
    Salon Products
Sea Minerals
Shaklee Corp.
ShiKai Products
Simmons Natural Bodycare
Smith & Vandiver
Soap Factory
Sombra Cosmetics
Swan Lake Botanicals
TerrEssentials
Tomé Professional Products
Tom's of Maine
Tova Corp.

Wachters' Organic Sea
    Products Corp.
Weleda
Wella Corporation
WiseWays Herbals
Wysong Corp.
Yves Rocher

HAIR COLORING
Alvin Last
American Int'l Ind.
Beauty Naturally
Chuckles
Colora Henna
Earth Science
JOICO Labs
Logona USA
Lotus Brands
Mastey De Paris
Mountain Rose Herbs
Nexxus Products
Rainbow Research Corp.
Revlon
Scruples Professional
    Salon Products
Starwest Botanicals
Wella Corporation

HAIR PERMS
ABBA Pure & Natural
    Hair Care
Beauty Naturally
Chuckles

John Paul Mitchell
    Systems
JOICO Labs
Mastey De Paris
Nexxus Products
Schwarzkopf & Dep
Scruples Professional
    Salon Products
Wella Corporation

INSECT REPELLENTS
Anthe-Essence
Aromatherapy
Appleberry Attic
Arbico Environmentals
Aroma Vera
Avon Products
Bi-O-Kleen Industries
Burt's Bees
Danklied Laboratories
Earth Science
Green Ban
Herb Garden
Herbal Products &
    Development
Heritage Store
Hummers
Kettle Care
Kyjen
Lakon Herbals
North Country
    Glycerine Soap
Safe Solutions

Simmons Natural
    Bodycare
Sunfeather Natural Soap
Swan Lake Botanicals
WiseWays Herbals

KITCHEN CLEANERS
ADWE Laboratories
Allens Naturally
Amazon Premium Products
American Eco-Systems
Arbico Environmentals
Aubrey Organics
Bath Island
Bio Pac
Bi-O-Kleen Industries
Body Crystal Environ-
    mental Products
Dial Corporation
Dr. Bronner's
    Magic Soaps
Earth Friendly Products
Earthly Matters
Espial USA
Faith Products
Hummers
Jelmar
McAuley's
NAACO
Natural Bodycare
Roebic Laboratories
Shadow Lake
Shaklee Corp.

Sierra Dawn Products
Simmons Natural
    Bodycare
Soap Factory
Sterling Clean
Unelko Corp.
Vermont Soapworks
Zenith Is 4 The Planet

LAUNDRY PRODUCTS

Allens Naturally
Amazon Premium
    Products
American Eco-Systems
Arbico Environmentals
Bio Pac
Bi-O-Kleen Industries
Dial Corporation
Earth Friendly Products
Espial USA
Faith Products
Frank T. Ross & Sons
Huish Detergents
Kleen Brite Labs
Lan-O-Sheen
Lifeline Company
NAACO
Natural Bodycare
Seventh Generation
Shadow Lake
Shaklee Corp.
Sierra Dawn Products

Simmons Natural
    Bodycare
Soap Factory
Soap Works
Sterling Clean
TerrEssentials
Vermont Soapworks
Wachters' Organic Sea
    Products Corp.
WiseWays Herbals
Zenith Is 4 The Planet

MASSAGE PRODUCTS

Abra Therapeutics
Ahimsa Natural Beauty
Alaska Herb & Tea
Alexandra Avery Purely
    Natural Body Care
Aloe Creme Laboratories
Alvin Last
Amrita Aromatherapy
Ancient Formulas
Anthe-Essence
Aromatherapy
Aphrodisia Products
Appleberry Attic
Aroma Life
Aroma Terra
Aroma Vera
Aromaland
Aubrey Organics
Avalon Natural Products

Bare Escentuals
Bath Island
Bavarian Alpenol &
    Sunspirit
Beehive Botanicals
Belle Star
Body & Soul
    Aromatherapy
Body Crystal Environ-
    mental Products
Body Tools
Bodyography
Borlind of Germany
Brookside Soap
Burt's Bees
CA-Botana Int'l
Catherine Atzen Laboratories
CD& P Health Products
Celestial Body
Chishti
Clarins of Paris
Colin Ingram
Earth Science
East End Imports
Elizabeth Van Buren
    Aromatherapy
Espial USA
Exotic Nature Body
    Care Products
Faith Products
Flower Essence Services
Freeman Cosmetic Corp.
Garden Botanika

Great Mother's Goods
Helen Lee Skin Care
  & Cosmetics
Herb Garden
Heritage Store
Indigo Wild Aromatics
Innovative Body Science
J & J Jojoba/California
  Gold Products
Jacki's Magic Lotion
Jason Natural Products
Kettle Care
Khepra Skin Care
Kim Manley Herbals
La Dove
Lakon Herbals
Lotus Brands
Lunar Farms Herbal
  Specialist
Maharishi Ayur-
  Veda Products
Mar-Riche Enterprises
Michael's Naturopathic
  Programs
Montagne Jeunesse
Motherlove herbal co.
Mountain Rose Herbs
Murad
Nadina's Cremes
Norimoor
Ohio Hempery
Penn Herb
Pharmagel Corp.

Prima Fleur Botanicals
Pure Touch Therapeutics
Rainbow Research Corp.
Rainforest
Ravenwood
Remington Products
Safe Solutions
Secret Gardens
Simmons Natural
  Bodycare
Smith & Vandiver
St. John's Herb Garden
Starwest Botanicals
Sumeru Garden Herbals
TerrEssentials
Tova Corp.
Uncommon Scents
V'tae Parfume &
  Body Care
Wachters' Organic Sea
  Products Corp.
Weleda
WiseWays Herbals
Yves Rocher

NAIL CARE

Abkit
Aloe Creme Laboratories
AM Cosmetics
American Int'l Ind.
Arizona Natural
  Resources
Aromaland

Avalon Natural
  Products
Bath & Body Works
Bodyography
Burt's Bees
CD&P Health
  Products
Clarins of Paris
Earth Science
Flowery Beauty Products
Focus 21 Int'l
Gap
Garden Botanika
Gena Laboratories
Honeybee Gardens
J. Stephen Scherer
Jackie Brown Cosmetics
Jafra Cosmetics Int'l
Jamieson Laboratories
Kettle Care
Khepra Skin Care
KSA Jojoba
Limited
Lotus Brands
Mar-Riche Enterprises
Mary Kay Cosmetics
Merle Norman Cosmetics
NaturElle Cosmetics
OPI Products
Pharmagel Corp.
Revlon
Tova Corp.
Vin-Dotco

WiseWays Herbals
Yves Rocher

PAPER PRODUCTS

Gillette
Herb Garden
Marcal Paper Mills
Ohio Hempery
Prima Fleur Botanicals
Seventh Generation
Vin-Dotco

PLANT CARE

Flower Essence Services
Mia Rose Products
St. Clair Industries
Wachters' Organic Sea
  Products Corp.
WiseWays Herbals
Wysong Corp.

POTPOURRI/ SACHETS/INCENSE

Alaska Herb & Tea
Aphrodisia Products
Appleberry Attic
Aroma Terra
Auroma Int'l
Bare Escentuals
Bath & Body Works
Bath Island
Belle Star
Body & Soul Aromatherapy

Body Tools
Chishti
Clear Light The Cedar Co.
Earth Science
Flower Essence Services
Gap
Garden Botanika
Helen Lee Skin Care
  & Cosmetics
Herb Garden
Heritage Store
Innovative Body Science
Kettle Care
Lotus Brands
McAuley's
Native Scents
Prima Fleur Botanicals
Pure Touch Therapeutics
Ravenwood
Sarah Michaels
Secret Gardens
Smith & Vandiver
St. John's Herb Garden
Starwest Botanicals
Surrey
Tova Corp.

SHAVING PRODUCTS

Alexandra Avery Purely
  Natural Body Care
Aloe Creme Laboratories
Alvin Last

American Int'l Ind.
American Safety Razor
Aroma Terra
Aubrey Organics
Avalon Natural
  Products
Bare Escentuals
Bath Island
Biogime Int'l
Body Crystal Environ-
  mental Products
Bodyography
Burt's Bees
CA-Botana Int'l
Clarins of Paris
Cold Wax
Derma E
Earth Science
Espial USA
Garden Botanika
Gillette
H2O Plus
Honeybee Gardens
Innovative Body
  Science
Izy's Aromatherapy
  Skin Care &
  Holistic Cosmetics
Jamieson Laboratories
Jason Natural Products
Kettle Care
Kiehl's
Kim Manley Herbals

KSA Jojoba
Les Femmes
Logona USA
Marilyn Miglin L.P.
Mar-Riche Enterprises
Mary Kay Cosmetics
Pharmagel Corp.
Prima Fleur Botanicals
Remington Products
Simmons Natural Bodycare
Smith & Vandiver
Surrey
TerrEssentials
Tom's of Maine
Tova Corp.
Uncommon Scents
Vermont Soapworks
Weleda
Wysong Corp.

SKIN CARE
Abkit
Abra Therapeutics
Absolute Aloe Int'l.
Adra Natural Soap
ADWE Laboratories
Ahimsa Natural Beauty
Alexandra Avery Purely
    Natural Body Care
Allon Personal Care
Aloe Commodities
Aloe Complete
Aloe Creme Laboratories

Alvin Last
Amazon Premium
    Products
American Int'l Ind.
American Safety Razor
Amrita Aromatherapy
Aphrodisia Products
Arizona Natural
    Resources
Aroma Life
Aroma Terra
Aroma Vera
Aubrey Organics
Auroma Int'l
Avalon Natural Products
Avon Products
Aztec Secret
Bare Escentuals
Bath & Body Works
Bath Island
Beauty Naturally
Beehive Botanicals
Belle Star
Biogime Int'l
Body & Soul
    Aromatherapy
Body Crystal Environ-
    mental Products
Body Shop
Bodyography
Bonne Bell
Borlind of Germany
Botanical Products

Brookside Soap
Burt's Bees
C.E. Hinds
CA-Botana Int'l
California Baby
    Botanical Skin Care
Catherine Atzen Labs
CD& P Health Products
Celestial Body
Chishti
Chuckles
Clarins of Paris
Classic Cosmetics
Clientele
Creme de la Terre
Deodorant Stones of
    America (D.S.A.)
Derma E
Derma-Life Corp.
Dial Corporation
Dreamous Corp.
East End Imports
Elizabeth Van Buren
    Aromatherapy
Espial USA
Estee Lauder Companies
Exotic Nature Body
    Care Products
Faith Products
Flower Essence Services
Freeman Cosmetic Corp.
Gabriel Cosmetics
Gap

Garden Botanika
Gena Laboratories
Gillette
H2O Plus
Helen Lee Skin Care
    & Cosmetics
Herb Garden
Herbal Products &
    Development
Heritage Store
Hobe Laboratories
Honeybee Gardens
Indigo Wild Aromatics
Innovative Body Science
Institute of Trichology
Izy's Aromatherapy
    Skin Care & Holistic
    Cosmetics
J & J Jojoba/California
    Gold Products
Jacki's Magic Lotion
Jafra Cosmetics Int'l
Jamieson Laboratories
Jason Natural Products
Jelene
JOICO Labs
Kettle Care
Khepra Skin Care
Kim Manley Herbals
Kiss My Face Corp.
KSA Jojoba
La Crista
La Dove

La Prairie
Lady of the Lake
Lakon Herbals
Levlad/Nature's Gate
Lily of Colorado
Limited
Logona USA
Lotus Brands
Lunar Farms Herbal
    Specialist
Magic of Aloe
Maharishi Ayur-Veda
    Products
Margarite Cosmetics/
    Moon Products
Marilyn Miglin L.P.
Mar-Riche Enterprises
Mary Kay Cosmetics
Mastey De Paris
McAuley's
Mera Personal Care Products
Merle Norman Cosmetics
Michael's Naturopathic
    Programs
Montagne Jeunesse
Mountain Ocean
Mountain Rose Herbs
Murad
Nadina's Cremes
Native Scents
Natural Bodycare
Natural Nectar Corp.
NaturElle Cosmetics

Nature's Radiance
Nature's Sunshine Products
Neo Tech Cosmetic
New Chapter
Nirvana
Nitro Stages Jolt
Norimoor
North Pacific Naturals
Nutri-Cell
Ohio Hempery
Orlane
Para Laboratories
Penny Island Products
Person & Covey
Pharmagel Corp.
Prima Fleur Botanicals
Pure Touch Therapeutics
Rainbow Research Corp.
Rainforest
Real Aloe
Redmond Minerals
Reviva Labs
Revlon
Rexall Showcase Int'l
Safe Solutions
Sappo Hill Soapworks
Sarah Michaels
Schwarzkopf & Dep
Scruples Professional
    Salon Products
Sea Minerals
Shaklee Corp.
ShiKai Products

Smith & Vandiver
Soap Factory
Soap Works
Sombra Cosmetics
St. Clair Industries
Starwest Botanicals
Sumeru Garden Herbals
Swan Lake Botanicals
TaUT by Leonard
  Engelman
TCCD Int'l
TerrEssentials
Tova Corp.
Uncommon Scents
Vermont Soapworks
Victoria's Secret
V'tae Parfume &
  Body Care
Wachters' Organic Sea
  Products Corp.
Weleda
WiseWays Herbals
Wysong Corp.
Yves Rocher
Zenith Is 4 The Planet
Zia Natural Skincare

Aubrey Organics
Avalon Natural
  Products
Avon Products
Azida
Bare Escentuals
Bath & Body Works
Bath Island
Bonne Bell
Borlind of Germany
CA-Botana Int'l
California Baby
  Botanical Skin Care
Catherine Atzen
  Laboratories
Clarins of Paris
Clientele
Derma-Life Corp.
Espial USA
Faith Products
Gabriel Cosmetics
Gap
Garden Botanika
H2O Plus
Heritage Store
Innovative Body
  Science
Island Dog
J & J Jojoba/California
  Gold Products
Jason Natural Products
Jelene
Kettle Care

Kiehl's
La Prairie
Levlad/Nature's Gate
Logona USA
Magic of Aloe
Mar-Riche Enterprises
Mary Kay Cosmetics
Mastey De Paris
Mountain Ocean
NaturElle Cosmetics
Nature's Sunshine
  Products
North Country
  Glycerine Soap
Person & Covey
Pharmagel Corp.
Prima Fleur Botanicals
Reviva Labs
Rexall Showcase Int'l
Safe Solutions
Simmons Natural
  Bodycare
Smith & Vandiver
St. Clair Industries
TaUT by Leonard
  Engelman
Terrapin Outdoor
  Systems
TerrEssentials
Tova Corp.
Wysong Corp.
Yves Rocher
Zia Natural Skincare

SUNSCREEN
Abra Therapeutics
Alexandra Avery Purely
  Natural Body Care
Aloe Creme Laboratories
Aroma Terra

♥ List of Cruelty-Free ♥ Mail-Order Companies

For your convenience, we have provided a listing of companies who provide mail-order service, in order to assist individuals who are having a difficult time finding particular items through stores in their area. Please refer to the product listing section on page 155 to help determine which companies sell particular products.

ABEnterprises
247 W. 38th St.
New York, NY 10018
(212)997-2307
Personal care, Household

Adrien Arpel
307 Treeworth Blvd.
Broadview Heights, OH 44147
(440)717-0860
Personal care, Cosmetics

Alaska Herb & Tea Co.
6710 Weimer Dr.
Anchorage, AK 99502
(907)245-3499
Personal care

Alexandra Avery Purely Natural Body Care
4717 SE Belmont
Portland, OR 97215
(800)669-1863
Personal care

Allens Naturally
P.O. Box 514, Dept. T
Farmington, MI 48332
(800)352-8971
Household

Allon Personal Care Corp.
25655 Springbrook Ave.
Saugus, CA 91350
(661)253-2723
Personal care

Aloe Creme Labs.
335 New Road
Monmouth Junction, NJ 08852-2311
(800)327-4969
Personal care, Cosmetics

Amazon Premium Products
275 NE 59th St.
Miami, FL 33137
(800)832-5645
Personal care, Cosmetics, Household, Companion animal

Amberwood
Route 2, Box 300, Baker County
Leary, GA 31762
(912)792-6246
Personal care, Cosmetics, Household, Companion animal

Aphrodisia Products, Inc.
62 Kent St.
Brooklyn, NY 11222
(718)383-3677
Personal care

Appleberry Attic
P.O. Box 135361
Clermont, FL 34713
(800)633-2682
Personal care, Companion animal

Arbico Environmentals
P.O. Box 4247
Tucson, AZ 85738
(520)825-9785
*Personal care, Cosmetics,
Household, Companion
animal*

Aroma Terra
P.O. Box 83027
Phoenix, AZ 83071
(800)456-3765
Personal care

AromaTherapeutix
P.O. Box 2908
Seal Branch, CA 90740
(800)308-6284
Personal care

Auromere Ayurvedic
Imports
2621 West Hwy. 12
Lodi, CA 95242
(800)735-4691
Personal care, Cosmetics

Avalon Natural Products
P.O. Box 750428
Petaluma, CA 94975
(707)769-5120
Personal care, Cosmetics

Ayurveda Holistic
Center
82A Bayville Ave.
Bayville, NY 11709
(516)628-8200
Companion animal

Back to Nature, Inc.
5627 N. Milwaukee Ave.
Chicago, IL 60646
(773)583-0402
*Personal care, Cosmetics,
Household, Companion
animal*

Bare Escentuals
600 Townsend St.
Ste. 329 East
San Francisco, CA 94103
(800)227-3990
Personal care, Cosmetics

Basically Natural
109 East G St.
Brunswick, MD 21716
(800)352-7099
*Personal care, Cosmetics,
Household, Companion
animal*

Beauty Naturally, Inc.
P.O. Box 4905
Burlingame, CA 94010
(650)697-1809
Personal care

Beehive Botanicals Inc.
Box 8257
Hayward, WI 54843
(800)283-4274
Personal care

Belle Star, Inc.
23151 Alcalde Dr., Ste. A-1
Laguna Hills, CA 92653
(949)768-7006
Personal care

Biogime Int'l, Inc.
25602 IH-45 North Fwy.
Spring, TX 77386
(800)338-8784
Personal care

Blessed Herbs
109 Barre Plains Rd.
Oakham, MA 01068
(508)882-3839
Personal care

Blue Ribbons Pet Care
1442 Peters Blvd.
Bay Shore, NY 11706
(800)552-BLUE
Companion animal

Body & Soul of Chicago
212 N. Shore Dr.
Oakwood Hills, IL 60013
(800)272-7085
Personal care

Body Encounters
604 Manor Rd.
Cinnaminson, NJ
08077
(800)839-2639
Personal care

The Body Shop
5036 One World Way
Wake Forest, NC 27587
(919)554-4900
Personal care, Cosmetics

Body Time
1101 Eighth St. Ste. 100
Berkeley, CA 94710
(510)524-0216
Personal care

Body Tools
16 Pamaron Way, Ste. C
Novato, CA 94949
(415)382-1355
Personal care

Bodyography
1641 16th St.
Santa Monica, CA 90404
(310)399-2886
Personal care, Cosmetics

C.E. Hinds
300 Wildwood Ave.
Woburn, MA 01801
(800)874-4788
Personal care, Cosmetics

Canada's All Natural
Soap, Inc.
P.O. Box 64567
Unionville, Ontario
L3R 0M9, Canada
(905)415-1540
*Personal care,
Companion animal*

Catherine Atzen
Laboratories
1790 Hamilton Ave.
San Jose, CA 95125
(800)468-4362
Personal care, Cosmetics

Celestial Body
21298 Pleasant Hill Rd.
Boonville, MO 65233
(800)882-6858
Personal care

Change of Face Cosmetics
P.O. Box 592
Hobart, IN 46342
(800)865-1755
Personal care, Cosmetics

Clear Conscience, LLC
P.O. Box 17855
Arlington, VA 22216
(800)595-9592
Personal care

Clear Light The Cedar Co.
Box 551 - State Rd. 165
Placitas, NM 87043
(800)557-3463
*Personal care, Cosmetics,
Household*

Color My Image Inc.
5025B Backlick Rd.
Annadale, VA 22003
(703)354-9797
Cosmetics

Common Scents
128 Main St.
Port Jefferson, NY 11777
(516)473-6370
Personal care

Cosmetique, Inc.
P.O. Box 94061
Palatine, IL 60094
(800)621-8822
Personal care, Cosmetics

Creme de la Terre
30 Cook Rd.
Stamford, CT 06902
(800)260-0700
Personal care

Dr. Goodpet
P.O. Box 4489
Inglewood, CA 90309
(800)222-9932
Companion animal

Dr. Hauschka Cosmetics
59C North St.
Hatfield, MA 01038
(413)247-9907
Personal care, Cosmetics

Dreamous Corp.
12016 Wilshire Blvd.
Los Angeles, CA 90025
(310)442-8544
Personal care, Cosmetics

Earth Doctor Distributor
828 Kings Rd.
Schenectady, NY 12303
(518)370-1904
Personal care, Household

East End Imports, Co.
47 North Shore Rd.
P.O. Box 107
Montauk, NY 11954
(516)668-4158
Personal care

EB5 Corp.
2232 E. Burnside St.
Portland, OR 97214
(503)230-8008
Cosmetics

Eco-Dent Int'l, Inc.
3130 Spring St.
Redwood City, CA
94063
(415)364-6343
Personal care

Eva Jon Cosmetics
1016 East California St.
Gainesville, TX 76240
(817)668-7707
*Personal care, Cosmetics,
Companion animal*

Everybody Ltd.
5150 Valmont Rd.
Boulder, CO 80301
(800)748-5675
Personal care

Exotic Nature Body
Care Products
2535 Village Lane, Ste. E
Cambria, CA 93428
(805)927-2517
Personal care

Fleabusters/Rx for Fleas,
Inc.
6555 NW 9th Ave.
Ft. Lauderdale, FL 33309
(800)666-3532
Companion animal

Flower Essence Services
P.O. Box 1769
Nevada City, CA 95959
(800)548-0075
*Personal care,
Companion animal*

For Pet's Sake
Enterprises, Inc.
3780 Eastway Rd.
Cleveland, Ohio 44118
(800)285-0298
Personal care, Cosmetics,

Gaiam Inc.
360 Interlocken Blvd.
Ste. 300
Broomfield, CO 80021
(800)869-3446
*Personal care, Cosmetics,
Household*

Garden Botanika
8624 154th Ave., N.E.
Redmond, WA 98052
(800)968-7842
Personal care, Cosmetics

Great Mother's Goods
501 West Fayette St.
Ste. 215
Syracuse, NY 13204
(315)476-1385
Personal care

Helen Lee Skin Care &
Cosmetics
205 East 60th St.
New York, NY 10022
(800)288-1077
Personal care, Cosmetics

Herb Garden
P.O. Box 773-N
Pilot Mountain, NC 27041
abeall@advi.net
Personal care, Household

Heritage Store, Inc.
314 Laskin Rd.
Virginia Beach, VA 23451
(800)TO-CAYCE
*Personal care, Cosmetics,
Household*

Home Service Products Co.
P.O. Box 129
Lambertville, NJ 08530
(609)397-8674
Household

Honeybee Gardens
P.O. Box 13
Morgantown, PA 19543
(888)478-9090
Personal care

Indigo Wild Aromatics
6503 Summit
Kansas City, MO 64113
(800)361-5686
*Personal care,
Companion animal*

Internatural
33719 116th
Twin Lakes, WI 53181
(800)643-4221
*Personal care, Cosmetics,
Household*

Izy's Aromatherapy Skin
Care & Holistic Cosmetics
13399 Terry
Detroit, MI 48227
(313)836-2675
Personal care, Cosmetics

J & J Jojoba/California
Gold Products
7826 Timm Rd.
Vacaville, CA 95688
(707)447-1207
Personal care, Cosmetics

Janene Int'l, Inc.
8604 2nd Ave., #147
Silver Spring, MD 20910
(800)480-3153
Personal care

Kettle Care
6590 Farm to Market Rd.
Whitefish, MT 59937
(406)892-3294
Personal care, Household

Kiehl's
109 Third Ave.
New York, NY 10003
(212)677-3171
Personal care, Cosmetics

Lady of the Lake Co.
P.O. Box 7140
Brookings, OR 97415
(503)469-3354
Personal care

Lily of Colorado
P.O. Box 12471
Denver, CO 80212
(800)333-5459
Personal care, Cosmetics

Lotions & Potions
406 S. Rockford Dr.
Tempe, AZ 85281
(800)462-7595
Personal care

Lotus Pads
131 NW Fourth, Ste. 156
Corvallis, OR 97330
503-758-4110
Personal care

Louise Bianco Skin Care
13655 Chandler Blvd.
Sherman Oaks, CA 91401
(800)782-3067
Personal care, Cosmetics

Magic of Aloe, Inc.
7300 N. Crescent Blvd.
Pennsauken, NJ 08110
(800)257-7770
Personal care, Cosmetics

Maharishi Ayur-Veda
Products
1068 Elkton Dr.
Colorado Springs, CO
80907
(719)260-5500
Personal care

Marilyn Miglin, L.P.
127 W. Huron
Chicago, IL 60610
(800)662-1120
Personal care, Cosmetics

Master's Flower Essences
14618 Tyler Foote Rd.
Nevada City, CA 95959
(800)347-3639
*Personal care,
Companion animal*

MDR Fitness Corp.
14101 N.W. Fourth St.
Sunrise, FL 33325
(954)845-9500
Personal care, Cosmetics

MediPatch Laboratories
Corp.
P.O. Box 795
E. Dennis, MA 02641
(508)385-4549
Companion animal

Mera Personal Care
Products
P.O. Box 218
Circle Pines, MN
55014
(800)752-7261
Personal care

Morrill's New Directions
21 Market Sq.
Houlton, ME 04730
(800)368-5057
*Personal care, Cosmetics,
Companion animal*

Motherlove Herbal
Company
P.O. Box 101
3101 Kintzley Plaza
Laporte, CO 80535
(970)493-2892
Personal care

Mountain Rose Herbs
20818 High St.
N. San Juan, CA 95960
(800)879-3337
*Personal care, Cosmetics,
Companion animal*

Nadina's Cremes
3813 Middletown
Branch Rd.
Vienna, MD 21869
(800)722-4292
Personal care, Cosmetics

Native Scents, Inc.
Box 5639
Toas, NM 87571
(800)645-3471
Personal care

Nature's Radiance
23704-5 El Toro Rd.,
PMB #513
Lake Forest, CA 92630
(877)628-8736
Personal care

Nature's WEALTH
2401 W. White Oaks Dr.
Springfield, IL 62704
(800)587-6288
Personal care

NaturElle Cosmetics Corp.
P.O. Box 3848
Telluride, CO 81435
(800)442-3936
Personal care, Cosmetics

Ohio Hempery
7002 St., Route 329
Guysville, OH 45735
(800)BUY-HEMP
Personal care

Paula's Choice -
Beginning Press
13075 Gateway Dr., #300
Tukwila, WA 98168
(800)831-4088
Personal care

Penn Herb Co., Ltd.
10601 Decatur Rd., Ste. 3
Philadelphia, PA 19154
(215)925-3336
Personal care

Philip B. Hair & Body Care
P.O. Box 15341
Beverly Hills, CA 90209
(800)643-5556
Cosmetics

Pickering & Simmons
2031 Route 130, Ste. D
Monmouth Junction, NJ
08852
Personal care

Precious Collection
Aromatherapy
P.O. Box 17155
Boulder, CO 80308
(800)877-6889
Personal care

Rainbow Research Corp.
170 Wilbur Pl.
Bohemia, NY 11716
(800)722-9595
Personal care

Rainforest Co.
141 Millwell Dr.
Maryland Heights, MO
63043
(314)344-1000
Personal care

Real Goods Trading Corp.
200 Clara Ave.
Ukiah, CA 95482
(707)468-9292
Personal care, Household

Rexall Showcase Int'l
851 Broken Sound
Pkwy., NW
Boca Raton, FL 33487
(800)327-0908
Personal care, Cosmetics

Schwarzkopf & Dep Inc.
2101 E. Via Arado Ave.
Rancho Dominguez, CA
90220
(800)367-2855
Personal care

Secret Gardens
P.O. Box B
Fall Creek, OR 97438
(800)537-8766
Personal care

Simmons Natural
Bodycare
42295 Hwy. 36
Bridgeville, CA 95526
(707)777-1920
*Personal care, Household,
Companion animal*

Simpler Thyme™
P.O. Box 2858
Branchville, NJ 07826
(973)875-9070
Personal care

Solid Gold Health
Products for Pets, Inc.
1483 N. Cuyamaca
El Cajon, CA 92020
(619)258-2780
Companion animal

Sombra Cosmetics Inc.
5600 - G McLeod, NE
Albuquerque, NM 87109
(800)225-3963
Cosmetics

St. John's Herb Garden
7711 Hillmeade Rd.
Bowie, MD 20720
(301)262-5302
Personal care

Steps In Health, Ltd.
P.O. Box 604426
Bayside, NY 11360
(800)471-VEGE
Personal care

Studio Magic, Inc.
20135-Cypress Creek Dr.
Alva, FL 33920
(941)728-3344
Personal care, Cosmetics

Sunfeather Natural Soap Co.
1551 Hwy. 72
Potsdam, NY 13676
(315) 265-3648
Personal care,
Companion animal

Swan Lake Botanicals
612 Dockery Lane
Mineral Bluff, GA
30559
(706)492-9927
Personal care, Cosmetics,
Companion animal

TaUT by Leonard
Engelman
9428 Eton, Ste. M
Chatsworth, CA 91311
(800)438-8288
Personal care, Cosmetics

TerrEssentials
2650 Old National Pike
Middletown, MD 21769
(301)371-7333
Personal care, Household,
Companion animal

Ultra Glow Cosmetics
P.O. Box 1469, Station A
Vancouver, BC
V6C 1P7, Canada
(604)444-4099
Personal care, Cosmetics

Uncommon Scents Inc.
380 W. 1st Ave.
Eugene, OR 97401
(800)426-4336
Personal care

Vanda Beauty Counselors
P.O. Box 3433
Orlando, FL 32802
(407)839-0223
Personal care, Cosmetics

Victoria's Secret Stores
P.O. Box 16586
Columbus, OH 43216
(614)856-6000
Personal care

Von Myering by Krystina
208 Seville Ave.
Pittsburgh, PA 15214
(412)766-3186
Personal care

Womankind
P.O. Box 1775
Sebastopol, CA 95473
(707)522-8662
Personal care

Wow-Bow Distributors
13 B Lucon Dr.
Deer Park, NY 11729
(800)326-0230
Companion animal

Yves Rocher, Inc.
491 John Young Way, #300
Exton, PA 19341-2548
(800)321-YVES
Personal care, Cosmetics

Zelda's
160 Esopus Ave.
Kingston, NY 12401
(800)647-8202
Personal care

Zenith Is 4 The Planet
P.O. Box 1739
Corvallis, OR 97339
(800)547-2741
Personal care, Household

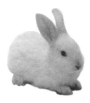

Companies That Did Not Respond to the NAVS Questionnaire

Questionnaires were sent to nearly 1000 companies at the beginning of our research for this book. The initial questionnaire was followed up by faxes and then telephone calls to try to obtain information from as many companies as possible. The following companies did not respond to the questionnaire. Inclusion in this section, however, is not necessarily an indication that a particular company conducts tests on animals. For further information, it is recommended that you contact the company directly. If you do receive information on a company's animal-testing policy, please let us know so that we can follow up with that company and pass on the information to readers in the future.

Addventure Products
5830 Oberlin Dr.
San Diego, CA 92121

Alpha 9
7400 E. Tierra Buena Ln.
Scottsdale, AZ 85260

Amole' Inc.
354 Ludlow Ave.
Cincinnati, OH 45220

Andrew Jergens Co.
2535 Spring Grove Ave.
Cincinnati, OH 45214

BeautiControl Cosmetics
2121 Midway Rd.
Carrollton, TX 75006

Beiersdorf, Inc.
360 Martin Luther King Dr.
Norwalk, CT 06856-5529

Bella's Secret Garden
P.O. Box 3994
Westlake, CA 93003

Benckiser Consumer
Products, Inc.
Five American Ln.
Greenwich, CT 06831

BeneFit Cosmetics
333 Kearny St., Ste. 200
San Francisco, CA 94108

Benjamin Ansehl Co.
1555 Page Industrial Blvd.
St. Louis, MO 63132

Bio-Tec Cosmetics Ltd.
92 Sherwood Ave.
Toronto, Ontario
M4P 2A7, Canada

BioFilm, Inc.
3121 Scott St.
Vista, CA 92083

Bissell, Inc.
2345 Walker, NW
Grand Rapids, WI 49544

Blue Coral, Inc.
5300 Harvard Ave.
Cleveland, OH 44105

Botanicus Inc.
7610 Rickenbacker Dr.
Gaithersburg, MD 20879

Breezy Balms
P.O. Box 588
Soquel, CA 95073

Brucci
861 Nepperham Ave.
Yonkers, NY 10703

Caraloe, Inc.
P.O. Box 168128
Irving, TX 75016

Caribbean Pacific
of the Rockies
P.O. Box 380
Crawford, CO 81415

Carme' Cosmeceutical
Sciences, Inc.
620 Airpark Rd.
Napa, CA 94558

Carter-Wallace, Inc.
1345 Ave. of the Americas
New York, NY 10105

Cassini Parfums, Ltd.
3 West 57th St., 8th Fl.
New York, NY 10019

Caswell-Massey
121 Fieldcrest Ave.
Edison, NJ 08818

Century Systems
120 Selig Dr., SW
Atlanta, GA 30336

Chattem, Inc.
1715 W. 38th St.
Chattanooga, TN 37409

Christian Dior Perfumes
9 W. 57th St., 39th Fl.
New York, NY 10019

Clean Brite Laboratories
4404 Anderson Dr.
Eau Claire, WI 54703

ClearVue Products, Inc.
P.O. Box 567
Lawrence, MA 01842

Color & Herbal Co.
4215 McEwen Rd.
Dallas, TX 75244

Comare Products
5980 Miami Lakes Dr.
Hialeah, FL 33014

Combe, Inc.
1101 Westchester Ave.
White Plains, NY 10604

ConAgra Pet Products
1 Century Park Plaza
Omaha, NE 68102-1675

Conair Corp.
1 Cummings Point Rd.
Stamford, CT 06904

Cooper Laboratories, Inc.
1132 Mark Ave.
Carpinteria, CA 93013

Cosmo Cosmetics, Inc.
10455 Slusher Dr.
Santa Fe Springs, CA 90670

Coty, Inc.
237 Park Ave., 9th Fl.
New York, NY 10017

Crabtree & Evelyn, Ltd.
P.O. Box 167
Woodstock, CT 06281

Creation Herbal Products
Route 1, Box 278
Blowing Rock, NC 28605

Creations Aromatiques
400 Sylvan Ave.
Englewood Cliffs, NJ 07632

Crowne Royale Ltd.
P.O. Box 5238
99 BRd. St.
Phillipsburg, NJ 08865

Crystal Companies
of California
10877 Wilshire Blvd., Los
Angeles, CA 90024

Crystalline Cosmetics
8436 N. 80th Pl.
Scottsdale, AZ 85258

Dental Herb Co., Inc.
78 Main St., P.O. Box 687
Northampton, MA 01061

Dermalogica, Inc.
1001 Knox St.
Torrance, CA 90502

Dermatologic Cosmetic
Laboratories
20 Commerce St.
East Haven, CT 06512

Desert Essence
9700 Topanga Canyon Blvd.
Chatsworth, CA 91311

Diamond Brands, Inc.
1660 South Hwy. 100
Minneapolis, MN 55416

Dionis Inc.
Post Office Box 5142
Charlottesville, VA 22905

Doak Dermatologics
383 Route 46 West
Fairfield, NJ 07004

Drs. Foster & Smith
2253 Air Park Rd.
Rhinelander, WI 54501

Dry Creek Herb Farm
13935 Dry Creek Rd.
Auburn, CA 95602

Earth Friendly Baby
P.O. Box 400
Charlotte, CT 05445

Earth Solutions, Inc.
1123 Zonolite, Ste. 8
Atlanta, GA 30306

Eden Botanicals
403 Laurel Glen Rd.
Soquel, CA 95073

Enesco Group Inc.
225 Windsor Dr.
Itasca, IL 60143

ES Laboratories
19417 63rd Ave. NE
Arlington, WA 98223

Essential Aromatics
205 N. Signal St.
Ojai, CA 93023

Essential Elements
2675 Folsom St.
San Francisco, CA 94110

Essential Products
of America, Inc.
8702 N. Mobley Rd.
Odessa, FL 33556

Essentially Yours
Industries Corp.
#201-8322 130th St.
Surrey, British Columbia
V3W-8J9 Canada

Fashion Fair Cosmetics
820 S. Michigan
Chicago, IL 60605

Faultless Starch/Bon Ami
1025 West 8th St.
Kansas City, MO 64101

Finelle Cosmetics c/o
Jeunique Int'l
P.O. Box 1950
City of Industry, CA 91749

Florida Pet Products, Inc.
P.O. Box 8631
Coral Springs, FL 33075

Focus 21 Int'l, Inc.
2755 Dos Aarons Way
Vista, CA 92083

Forest Essentials
601 Del Norte Blvd.
Oxnard, CA 93030

Fort James Corp.
P.O. Box 19130
Green Bay, WI 54307

Fruit of the Earth, Inc.
P.O. Box 152044
Irving, TX 75015-2044

Fuller Brush Co.
P.O. Box 1247
Great Bend, KS 67530

Glo-Marr Products, Inc.
400 Lincoln St.
Lawrenceburg, KY 40342

Glover Hair Products
1645 Oak St.
Lakewood, NJ 08701

Gold Shield
P.O. Box 858
Mahwah, NJ 07430

Golden Star, Inc.
400 East Tenth Ave.
N. Kansas City, MO 64116

Goldwell Cosmetics (USA)
981 Corporate Blvd.
Linthicum Heights, MD
21090

Grace Cosmetics
#120 6330 12th St. SE
Calgary, Alberta
T2H 2X2, Canada

Guerlain, Inc.
444 Madison Ave.
New York, NY 10022

Guthy-Renker Corp.
41-550 Eclectic
Palm Desert, CA 92260

Hazel Bishop Int'l
910 Sylvan Ave.
Englewood Cliffs, NY 07632

Healthy Times
13200 Kirkham Way
Poway, CA 92064

Hermes of Paris, Inc.
745 Fifth Ave., #800
New York, NY 10151

Holloway House Inc.
P.O. Box 50126
Indianapolis, IN 46250

Home Health
90 Orville Dr.
Bohemia, NY 11716

Hygenic Cosmetics, Inc.
6500 NW Twelfth Ave.
Ft. Lauderdale, FL 33309

Il-Makiage Inc.
45-49 Davis St.
Long Island City, NY 11101

Image Laboratories, Inc.
1850 N. McNab Rd.
Ft. Lauderdale, FL 33309

IQ Products Co.
16212 State Hwy. 249
Houston, TX 77086

J. F. Lazartigue
764 Madison Ave.
New York, NY 10021

Janca's Jojoba Oil
& Seed Co.
456 East Juanita, #7
Mesa, AZ 85204

Janet Sartin Cosmetics
500 Park Ave.
New York, NY 10022

Jessica McClintock
1400 Sixteenth St.
San Francisco, CA 94103

Joe Blasco Cosmetic Co.
7340 Greenbriar Pkwy.
Orlando, FL 32819

Johnson Products Co.
8522 S. Lafayette Ave.
Chicago, IL 60620

Jojoba Resources, Inc.
P.O. Box 6513
Chandler, AZ 85246

Just for Redheads
115 Juniper Trail
Sedona, AZ 86336

Juvenesse by Elaine Gayle
680 N. Lake Shore Dr.
Chicago, IL 60611

Kama Sutra Co.
2260 Townsgate Rd.
Westlake Village, CA 91361

Katonah Scentral
51 Katonah Ave.
Katonah, NY 10536

Key Distributors, Inc.
16035 East Arrow Hwy.
Irwindale, CA 91706

Kirkland Signatures
P.O. Box 34535
Seattle, WA 98124

KIT Products
2545-A Prairie Rd.
Eugene, OR 97402

Kiwi Brands
447 Old Swede Rd.
Douglassville, PA 19518

L'Herbier De Provence
462 Fashion Ave., Fl. 17
New York, NY 10018

Lambert-Kay
Research Way
P.O. Box 1418
Princeton, NJ 08512

Laura Mercier
2900 Weslayan, Ste. 415
Houston, TX 77027

Lily of the Desert
1887 Geesling Rd.
Denton, TX 76208

Lime-O-Sol
101 S. Parker Dr.
State Rd. 4
Ashley, IN 46705

LVMH Moet Hennessy
Louis Vuitton
30 Avenue Hoche
F-75008 Paris, France

Marae Storm
P.O. Box 203
Branscomb, CA 95417

Masada Marketing Co.
P.O. Box 4118
Chatsworth, CA 91313

Menley & James Labs
125 Strafford Ave.
Wayne, PA 19087-3337

Micro Balanced Products
225 County Rd.
Tenafly, NJ 07670

Most Products Inc.
326 W. Kalamazoo Ave.
Kalamazoo, MI 49007

Nature's Fresh Northwest
3008 SE Division
Portland, OR 97202

NeoStrata Co.
4 Research Way
Princeton, NJ 08540

Neoteric Cosmetics
4880 Havana St.
Denver, CO 80239

New Dana Perfumes
3 Landmark Sq.
Stamford, CT 06901

Oasis Brand Products
P.O. Box 12871
La Jolla, CA 92039

One World Botanicals
6 E. Washington Ave.
Atlantic Highlands, NJ
07716

Orjene Natural Cosmetics
543 48th Ave.
Long Island City, NY 11101

Paco Rabanne Parfums
70 East 55th St., 17th Fl.
New York, NY 10022

Parfums Givenchy, Inc.
717 Fifth Ave.
New York, NY 10022

Parker & Bailey
141 Middle St.
Portland, ME 04101

Paul Mazzotta, Inc.
P.O. Box 96
Reading, PA 19607

Pet Tech, Inc.
7403 Lakewood Dr., W.
Tacoma, WA 98467

Pets 'N' People Inc.
27520 Hawthorne Blvd.
Palos Verdes Estates, CA
90274

Physicians Formula
1055 W. 8th St.
Azusa, CA 91702

Prestige Cosmetics
1441 W. Newport Center Dr.
Deerfield Beach, FL 33442

Principal Secret, c/o
Victoria Principal GRC
41550 Eclectic St.
Palm Desert, CA 92260

Procyte Corp.
8511 154th Ave. NE
Redmond, WA 98052

Quan Yin Essentials
P.O. Box 1050
Mt. Shasta, CA 96067

RAF Trading Corp.
95 W. 3rd St.
Freeport, NY 11520

Ranir Corp./DCP
P.O. Box 8547, 4701 E.
Paris Ave. SE
Grand Rapids, MI 49512

RC Int'l
11222 I. Street
Omaha, NE 68137

Rio Vista Products
P.O. Box 60806
Santa Barbara, CA 93160

Riviera Concepts, Inc.
150 Duncan Mill Rd.
Don Mills, Ontario
M3B 3M4 Canada

Sanofi Beaute, Inc.
90 Park Ave.
New York, NY 10019

Santa Fe Fragrance Inc.
P.O. Box 282
Santa Fe, NM 87504

Scandinavian Natural
Health & Beauty Products
13 N. Seventh St.
Perkasie, PA 18944

Schroeder & Tremayne
8450 Valcour
St. Louis, MO 63123

Shiseido Cosmetics
(America) Ltd.
900 Third Ave., 15th Fl.
New York, NY 10022

Silvestre
4319 Oak Lawn Ave.
Dallas, TX 75219

Simple Wisdom, Inc.
775 S. Graham
Memphis, TN 38111

Soft Sheen Products, Inc.
1000 E. 87th St.
Chicago, IL 60619

Strickland, J. & Co.
P.O. Box 840
Memphis, TN 38101

Susan Lucci Hair Care
505 S. Beverly Dr.
Beverly Hills, CA 90210

Talisman
410 E. Denny Way
Seattle, WA 98122

Tender Corp.
P.O. Box 290
Littleton, NH 03561

Tiffany & Co.
727 Fifth Ave.
New York, NY 10022

Trader Joe's Co.
538 Mission St.
S. Pasadena, CA 91030

Tressa, Inc.
P.O. Box 75320
Cincinnati, OH 45275

Tropix Suncare Products
1014 Laurel St.
Brainerd, MN 56401

Tsumura Int'l
300 Lighting Way, 6th Fl.
Secaucus, NJ 07096

Twincraft
2 Tigan St.
Winooski, VT 05404

Urban Decay
2060 Placentia Ave.
Costa Mesa, CA 92627

Vapor Products
P.O. Box 56839
Orlando, FL 32586

Veterinarian's Best
P.O. Box 4459
Santa Barbara, CA 93103

Victoria Jackson Cosmetics
1230 American Blvd.
Westchester, PA 19380

ViJon Laboratories, Inc.
6300 Etzel Ave.
St. Louis, MO 63133

Virginia's Soap Ltd.
Group 60 Box 20
RR #1
Anola, Manitoba
R0E 0A0 Canada

Vital Health Products
8544 W. National Ave.
Milwaukee, WI 53227

Wally's Natural Products
P.O. Box 5275
Auburn, CA 95604

Watkins Inc.
150 Liberty St.
Winona, MN 55987

Wild Aster Farm
3756 Reamer Rd.
Lapeer, MI 48446

Wild Oats Corporation
1645 Broadway St.
Boulder, CO 80302

Wilkes Group, Inc.
7 Vista Dr.
Old Lyme, CT 06371

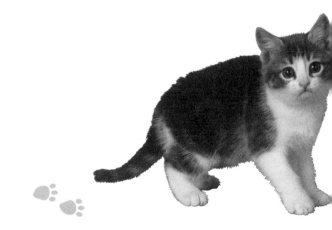

The National Anti-Vivisection Society:
Advocates for Humane Science

Founded in 1929 as a small group of dedicated individuals passionately opposed to the suffering of animals inflicted in the name of science, the National Anti-Vivisection Society (NAVS) has been dedicated to developing educational programs that promote *humane solutions to human problems.* Our mission is to end the use of animals in research, product testing and education through programs that educate the public about the cruelty and waste of vivisection and to encourage the development of non-animal methodologies.

With the help of our supporters, NAVS' credible and solution-oriented programs have helped to spare countless animals from needless suffering while promoting ethical and innovative scientific endeavors. We are proud to say that through our nationwide education programs, NAVS has played an instrumental role in changing the attitudes of people—both the general public and the scientific community—about the ethical issues and scientific arguments against vivisection.

Publications such as *Personal Care for People Who Care* have provided the public with the specific information needed to persuade many of the largest consumer companies to halt or dramatically reduce the testing of their products on animals. Working with other animal advocacy groups, NAVS' legal and legislative efforts have assisted in the passage of student choice bills allowing students to choose an alternative to dissection and enabled citizens to gain access to research records through freedom of information petitions. And working with dedicated scientists, we have been instrumental in proving that valid alternatives to the use of animals in research, product testing, and education can be developed.

In advancing credible solutions for a cruelty-free world, NAVS does not threaten medical progress. We are not anti-science. Our message is simple: animal research is not a solution. It's a problem—a costly problem in terms of animal lives and in terms of human health and progress towards medical cures.

Despite our progress, vivisection remains pervasive and we continue to need the support of compassionate individuals to ensure that our life-saving work can go on until this cruel and wasteful practice is completely abolished.

✔ The NAVS Dissection Hotline (**1-800-922-FROG**) is the only national toll-free counseling service which provides support to students, their parents and teachers who object to dissection and want to learn more about their options. This free service is helping to ensure that the next generation of scientists and health care professionals are encouraged to pursue their goals without harming animals. This is especially crucial at a time when elementary schools are increasing dissection exercises in their curriculum for younger students.

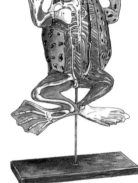

✔ The NAVS Dissection Alternatives Loan Program offers an extensive inventory of plastic animal models and interactive computer software to individual students and schools on a free loan basis. Students and teachers can use these tools to experience the wonder and mystery of biological processes without sacrificing their respect for life.

✔ NAVS provides financial support to the International Foundation for Ethical Research, which awards grants to scientists to develop viable alternatives to the use of animals in product testing, research and education. Grants are also available to postgraduate students who wish to incorporate animal welfare issues into their studies.

✔ NAVS advances justice for animals by putting the law to work for them. NAVS monitors and promotes legislation and participates in government rulemaking. NAVS has founded the International Institute for Animal Law to advance credible scholarship and advocacy skills within the legal community for the benefit of animal protection. AnimalLaw.com is in the forefront of providing legal resources for the benefit of animals via the internet, while the National Research Library for Animal Advocacy, founded by NAVS in cooperation with The John Marshall Law School in Chicago, offers a selection of published materials and a comprehensive bibliography of animal resources.

✔ In response to all too frequent emergency situations of animals in urgent need of assistance, NAVS has recently established a special Sanctuary Fund designed to provide timely financial assistance to animal organizations involved in emergency animal rescues.

Despite these efforts, we still have much to do. New challenges on the horizon, such as genetic engineering, cloning and transplanting animal parts into humans, threaten to use animals in ever more bizzare ways.

Please consider joining NAVS...and making a real difference for all the innocent animals who cannot speak for themselves. You'll find a membership application on page 193. Please make copies and give them to your friends who are also committed to bringing compassion, respect and justice to all living creatures.

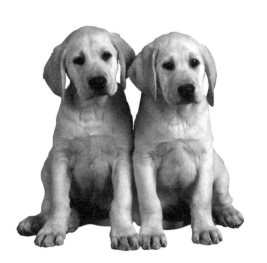

NAVS Membership Application

Please join us in our work to end animal suffering. Call (800)888-NAVS(6287) or mail this application today to NAVS, P.O. Box A3728, Chicago, IL 60690-9528.

I want to join the National Anti-Vivisection Society. I understand that my new membership includes one free copy of *Personal Care for People Who Care,* regular issues of the NAVS *Animal Action Report* and other important updates.

Please check all appropriate boxes below.

Annual Memberships
- ❐ Individual $25   P1N01
- ❐ Student $10   P1N06
- ❐ Senior $12   P1N05

Lifetime Memberships
- ❐ Life Sponsor $100   P1N04
- ❐ Life Benefactor $500   P1N02
- ❐ Life Partner $1,000   P1N03

❐ Please send me additional information on NAVS' programs.   P1G00

❐ I do not wish to join at this time, but please accept my donation of $ _____   P1010

❐ Please send me more information on how I can enjoy the convenience of having a monthly donation debited from my credit card, checking or savings account.   P1Z00

❐ My check is enclosed. Charge my   ❐ VISA   ❐ MasterCard   ❐ Discover

Account No. _____ Exp. Date _____

Signature _____

Telephone Number _____

Name _____

Address _____

City_____ State_____ Zip_____

Please do not send cash. All contributions are tax-deductible to the fullest extent allowed by law. If you are using a credit card, you may also FAX this application to NAVS at: (312)427-6524.

NOTES

NAVS Merchandise Order Form

ITEM	PRICE	QUANTITY	AMOUNT DUE
Books			
Lethal Laws (Fano)	$10.95		
Next of Kin (Roger Fouts/Stephen Tukel Mills)	$19.95		
Declaration of the Rights of Animals	$10.00		
Personal Care For People Who Care 10th Ed. (NAVS)	$9.50		
The Great Ape Project (Cavalieri & Singer)	$11.85		
Animals in Education (Hepner)	$11.65		
The Monkey Wars (Blum)	$15.00		
Why Do Vegetarians Eat Like That (Gabbe)	$8.40		
Of Mice, Models, and Men (Rowan)	$19.95		
Diet For A New America (Robbins)	$13.95		
The Cruel Deception (Sharpe)	$12.00		
Animal Liberation (Singer)	$12.95		
67 Ways To Save the Animals (Sequoia)	$4.95		
Dog Scrap Book	$1.00		
NAVS Co-Sponsored Books			
Alcoholic Rats	$3.95		
Maternal Deprivation	$4.95		
Heart Research	$4.95		
Cancer Research	$4.95		
Set of Four	$16.00		
Posters			
Declaration of the Rights of Animals (sm. poster)	$3.00		
Declaration of the Rights of Animals (lrg. poster)	$7.00		
Art for Animals Classic Poster: Still Life (cat)	$6.00		
Art for Animals Classic Poster: Research (chimp)	$6.00		
Art for Animals Classic Poster: Together (world)	$6.00		
Merchandise			
Art for Animals Classic Stickers (32 count)	$1.00		
Quotes of Compassion Stickers (32 count)	$1.00		
Compassionate Creatures Stickers (24 count)	$3.00		
"Laps Not Labs" Cat Stickers (32 count)	$1.00		
Quotes of Compassion Mug	$6.00		
"Respect Don't Dissect" Mug	$6.00		
"Respect, Don't Dissect" Frog Pencil	$1.25		
NAVS Chimp Notepads (25 sheets)	$1.00		
See back of this page for totaling/shipping information.	**SUBTOTAL**		

Continued on back

NAVS Merchandise Order Form—Continued

ITEM	PRICE	QUANTITY	AMOUNT DUE
T-shirts and Sweatshirts			
"Respect Don't Dissect" T-shirt (L or XL only)	$15.00		
"Have A Heart" T-shirt (L or XL only)	$15.00		
Global Awareness T-shirt (L or XL only)	$15.00		
"It Doesn't Take A Genius" Sweatshirt (M or L only)	$20.00		
Combined subtotal from previous page and this page: **AMOUNT DUE**			
Subtract 10% Member Discount			
Plus Shipping & Handling			
TOTAL			

Shipping & Handling Charges

Up to $5.99= $1.50
$6.00 - $11.99= $2.50
$12.00 - $17.99= $3.50
Each Add'l $6.00= $1.50

Credit Card: ☐ VISA ☐ MC ☐ Discover

Exp. Date _____

Account Number _____

Daytime Phone _____

Signature _____

NAME: _____

ADDRESS: _____

CITY/STATE/ZIP: _____

Shipping address if different than billing address:

_____

_____

Clip or photocopy this form and mail to: The National Anti-Vivisection Society, 53 W. Jackson Blvd., Ste. 1552, Chicago, IL 60604. Check, money order or credit card payment only. No cash. All contributions are tax-deductible to the fullest extent allowed by law.

NAVS Survey

We Need Your Feedback!

Please help us in our ongoing effort to keep *Personal Care for People Who Care* the most current and comprehensive book of its kind by filling out the following survey. Although we try, all products and companies may not be listed here so please let us know what you think might be missing. When completed, send the survey to:

The National Anti-Vivisection Society
53 W. Jackson Blvd., Suite 1552
Chicago, IL 60604

Thank you for your help!

Did you have any trouble finding the listings you were looking for?
❏ Yes ❏ No
If yes, explain.

_____

_____

Is there any other information you would like to see included in future editions of *Personal Care for People Who Care?*

_____

How did you find out about this book?

_____

Would you recommend this book to others?
❏ Yes ❏ No

(Please complete the other side of this survey) ⇨

If you have information about a company or product that was not included in this edition, please provide it here so that we can solicit information for the future. Providing an address and phone number will help speed up our inquiry. Check the product label, if you have it, for company information.

Company Name_____ Product Name _____
Address _____
City_____State_____ Zip_____
Telephone Number _____FAX Number _____

Company Name_____ Product Name _____
Address _____
City_____State_____ Zip_____
Telephone Number _____FAX Number _____

Company Name_____ Product Name _____
Address _____
City_____State_____ Zip_____
Telephone Number _____FAX Number _____

Company Name_____ Product Name _____
Address _____
City_____State_____ Zip_____
Telephone Number _____FAX Number _____

Are you a member of NAVS?
❒ Yes ❒ No

Thanks again for your feedback!

NOTES

NOTES